What the...?

I *Can't* Eat *THAT* Anymore?

Discovering a life without gluten and why a
simple diet switch is not what it seems

Jodie Clapp

ThinkHouse Publishing. PO Box 200 South Grafton, NSW, 2460 Australia

For information about special discounts available for bulk purchases, contact Jodie@thegfhub.com

Collaborators:

Kathleen Watson, Editor, Cypress Press LLC.
Sarah Chalmers, Proofreader.
Ana Voicu, Cover Designer.
Joel Ibarra, eBook Conversion Specialist.

Dedication

To all my fellow knowing and unknowing celiac and gluten-sensitive friends out there. This book is for you.

A big thank you to my family and friends for their support, for putting up with me talking about this damn book for years and a very special thank you, in particular, to my supportive man for surviving my rants, raves, dummy-spits, and tears. But most of all for giving me encouragement to write this book, the motivation to not give up, and the occasional kick up the butt needed to stay on track.

Table of Contents

The Serious Part

*L*et's talk about the elephant in the room.

I am not a doctor, qualified nutritionist, specialist, or medically trained in any way.

I am a geek who studies health and nutrition for a hobby. I learn from some of the best doctors around the world and spend my free time listening to podcasts, watching summits, and gorging myself on medical books. All the information in this book is from my years of research and personal experience as a patient of celiac disease and a patient of life. These are my views, opinions, and knowledge of what I've learned that I am sharing with you.

I am not giving anyone medical advice. I am not an expert, gastroenterologist, or microbiologist, but I do talk about these topics and the information I have found within them. My goal is to share with you my journey with celiac disease, my wins and losses, and deliver what I've learned along the way in a fun and entertaining manner.

Disclaimer

The information provided in this book is designed to provide helpful information on the subjects discussed. Information and statements made are not intended to replace the advice of your doctor. The author does not dispense medical advice, prescribe, or diagnose illness.

This book is not meant to be used, nor should it be used, to diagnose or treat any medical condition. For diagnosis or treatment of any medical problem, consult your own physician.

The author is not responsible for any specific health or allergy needs that may require medical supervision and is not liable for any damages or negative consequences from any treatment, action, application, or preparation to any person reading or following the information in this book.

It is sold with the understanding that the publisher is not engaged to render any type of psychological, medical, nutritional, or any other kind of professional advice.

References are provided for informational purposes only and do not constitute endorsement of any websites or other sources.

Readers should be aware that the websites listed in this book may change.

The views and nutritional information expressed are not intended to be a substitute for conventional medical service.

Introduction

If you're reading this book, perhaps you have noticed there might be something wrong going on inside your body. Do you suspect gluten is the culprit but don't know where to start?

Or perhaps you've been given the news that you're diagnosed with celiac disease and possibly feeling your life is about to change.

You may not believe me right now, but maybe by the end of this book, you'll come to the same realization I did: going gluten-free is really not that bad after all.

When I was first diagnosed, I picked up a loaf of gluten-free bread and read the ingredients. I was astounded at the chemical maze that made up this product I was about to consume. After some investigation of those ingredients, I realized a simple switch to gluten-free products was not going to help me lead a healthy life and might actually do harm in the long run. I decided right there and then that I was going to research and investigate gluten-free products and blow the whistle on what could be a potentially unhealthy lifestyle for many sufferers. I learned the negative effects that some gluten-free products can have on the body and how to find better quality options. In this book, I show you what those options look like and how to find them.

Over the years while I wrote this book, I figured out how to change my life *and* my thinking. They were probably some of my most challenging years yet. I have taken everything I've learned over my celiac journey—from science, to learning curves, to emotions, to discoveries—and have compiled it all into this book.

Hopefully, it's a book you can laugh at, cry at, maybe even throw across the room if you need to, but most of all, a book that may give you some answers, understanding, guidance, and possibly shine a new light on what might feel like— at least, right now—a pretty shitty and confusing situation.

My new passion in life is *The GF[1] Hub*, a website I'm building where us allergy sufferers, celiacs, gluten-sensitive, and health-conscious people can get together and share knowledge, recipes, events, and passion for living a new way of life. Head to www.thegfhub.com and sign up to our mailing list for updates and be involved as the site grows, but in the meantime, have some fun with the info on our site and get together with us on social platforms.

Please join me on:

- Thegfhub.com
- Facebook Page: The GF Hub
- Facebook Group: The Gluten-free Hub
- Instagram @thegfhub
- Twitter @thegfhub

I would love to hear your feedback and thoughts about my book. I'd be very grateful if you could leave a review on the place of purchase (Amazon, iBooks etc.), or simply email me directly at jodie@thegfhub.com with any other questions you may have. I love to chat, and you will know just how much by the end of this book!

---

[1] gluten-free

What the...!
I Can't Eat THAT Anymore?

I'm a true-blue Aussie girl. I wear thongs (aka flip-flops), drink beer at BBQs, and enjoy the Aussie lifestyle. I grew up on a country farm and moved to the suburbs on the eastern beaches of Queensland, Australia in my teens. Although I call Australia home, I've been lucky enough to travel to some pretty amazing countries around the world. To sum me up:

Adventure + Travel + Food = ME

Or so I thought. Life has a funny way of throwing you curveballs.

When gallivanting around the world I've been fortunate enough to sample some of the most sumptuous foods available. From gooey fondue in Switzerland to perfectly roasted Thanksgiving turkey in the USA, to cold raw chicken in Japan, and the list goes on. I once dragged my husband halfway across Sweden just to go to a particular restaurant I'd read about. When we arrived, he slowly nodded and gave me a half-real, half-I'm-going-to-kill-you smile when I asked, *"Do you like vegan?"*

I filled my days off from work with shuffling through the local newspapers in search of the next food festival and blogging about cafes and restaurants I visited.

I'm grateful to have a close friend who shares my love of food discovery. So much so, that when our local community Christmas Carol festival was on, we loaded up several bags filled with exotic cheeses, cured meats, fresh grapes, dried figs, quince paste, feta stuffed peppers, rustic French sourdough baguettes, delectable dips, and paired them all with three bottles of well-aged Italian Shiraz. We set off on our pushbikes to the event, carrying all our food and a super-sized picnic blanket looking like a couple of pack horses.

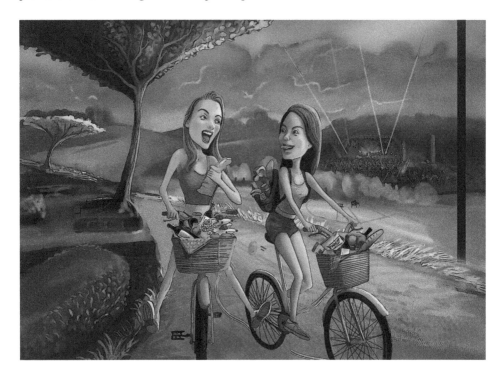

It was a hot, humid, summery Christmas night and we arrived early at the park, achieving a proud and prime location to set up what looked like a full-blown delicatessen, all laid out perfectly on our red and black-checkered blanket. We received some funny looks and comments throughout the night as we gorged ourselves fully, drank ourselves silly, then had a ton of fun trying to pedal our pushbikes home in the dark…pissed as farts and drunk as skunks.

Despite my love of food and wine, I've always exercised regularly and have always been a healthy eater. However, it was not uncommon on my cheat days or naughty nights to eat a pizza and slug back a few beers while watching the Formula 1 with my husband or *The Notebook* if I got my way. Some days I ate deep-fried fish and chips at the beach and others were filled with popcorn and ice-cream.

Just for fun, and much to my husband's frustration, in my exploration of food and health, I've tried many diet lifestyles like vegan, paleo, raw, blood type, etc. just to see what they were like. I was one of the lucky people who cruised through life with no adverse reactions to eating anything. I didn't have any food allergies or intolerances and I could eat all the pasta, breads, and grains I ever wanted without so much as letting off a fart. I thought I had a cast iron gut! So, it was the biggest surprise to me when a hematologist gave me the life-changing news:

"You have celiac disease!"

You might think, if you didn't get sick from eating food, then how did you end up at a hematologist getting a celiac disease diagnosis? There must have been something wrong.

And you're right, there was.

Let me start at the beginning.

Chapter 2

My Rant & Rave

As defined by the Oxford dictionary:
Rant and rave: To shout and complain angrily about something at length. Ok…so it won't be that bad. I promise!

Once a year, I get a full set of blood tests done to check all my levels.

I come from a family history of auto-immune diseases, heart disease, and cancer, so this was just my little control-freak thing I do to make sure I am always in good health and would not end up like my other family members. I treat myself like my own little human experiment in a way.

When it came to doctors reviewing these test results,[2] they only looked for the little **'L'** and **'H'** markers next to the test range to show 'Low' and 'High.' This flags if there is an issue with the levels. It seemed that, unless the doctor saw these markers, they looked no further and sent me on my way.

In the early part of 2013, I went to see the doctor about my recent test results. There was nothing to discuss as far as he was concerned but I requested a copy of the results so I could look for myself. I noticed my iron had dropped significantly lower than usual. It was right on the 'Low' borderline range but didn't flag the little 'L,' and sure enough, the doctor did not care to discuss this with me.

This drop in iron was unexpected as I hadn't changed my lifestyle or eating habits. It didn't seem like a good thing, so I took some supplements to see if they would help. I went back again the following year for the tests, and sure enough,

---

[2] Please note: This relates to Australian blood test results. I'm not sure how it works in other countries.

my iron had plummeted even further. Now it was below the bottom of the acceptable range.

This time it flagged the indicator because I was now anemic. I explained to my doctor I had noticed this drop the previous year and had been taking supplements to help, but now it was even lower again. His suggestion was to up the dosage of supplements and check again the following year. I thought a year was a long time to wait and see if it had any effect, especially considering I had already been taking supplements for a year already. But perhaps the body needed time to adjust and the doctor was the expert…right?

That following year, I circulated between every kind of iron pill, liquid, tonic, and powder I could find. I even tried combining iron with other vitamins like vitamin C to help with iron absorption.

The next year's tests came back and again it was worse. There was no change in sentiment or recommendations from the doctor on how to improve this situation. I even went to see a different doctor for another opinion, but that was of little help, as they didn't offer me any other suggestion except to keep taking more pills.

I spent hundreds and hundreds of dollars again the following year trying to get my iron up to no avail.

By the end of the third year, and with my third doctor, the results did not improve, and I was really getting disappointed as I felt like I was receiving no help or guidance from anyone. The doctors did not seem to be worried about my worsening condition, which gave me the feeling that I was being melodramatic.

Am I making a bigger deal out of it than what I should be? I thought. Surely not. Isn't anemia a very serious condition?

I was having the same feeling all over again. The same feeling I'd had when I was 25 years old and very sick with abdominal pain. At the time, I knew something was wrong but several doctors and ultrasound companies told me there was nothing wrong with me.

"It's all in your head," they said.

I persevered to find out what was going on, and within a very short period, I was in the hospital for a week, having a massive operation for an extreme case of endometriosis. I had 43 cysts removed from my bowels, bladder, and internal cavity, and they removed two lemon-sized cysts growing on each ovary.

So, it wasn't all in my head.

I didn't take *no* for an answer then; why should I now?

One might ask, "Why didn't you just Google low iron to figure it out yourself?"

Low iron can mean so many things. I didn't want to jump to conclusions as I would probably see the word *cancer* in there somewhere and absolutely crap my pants!

I called my gynecologist and asked if the pill I was taking to help control my endometriosis could cause my low iron levels. He genuinely took my situation and concern seriously and recommended I see a hematologist right away.

Well, that was a suggestion I could have done with a few years ago. Evidently, it sometimes pays to follow up with a specialist. I was so deeply disappointed that I'd had a run of bad luck with doctors not seeming to care or want to help. I felt like just a number in and out the door. But for me, this was my life. I'm sure there are some amazing doctors out there and at least now I hoped I was on the right path.

To see a specialist, you need a doctor's referral, so I made an appointment to see a local doctor and explained my iron history issues and that I wanted to see a hematologist. He asked if I had been getting sick from food and my answer was no. That was the truth. I noticed his referral said, *"No symptoms suggestive of celiac disease."* So it would seem that because I didn't get sick from food, there was no need to test for anything or look further into the matter?

I made the appointment to see the hematologist and explained my scenario. I showed her all my blood work over the years, pre-and post-iron drop in 2013. I explained my efforts with supplements had no positive effect. I expressed my concerns with sheer desperation in hope that she would help. I wanted someone to take me—and my situation—seriously for once.

She confirmed I was anemic and ordered me to go to the hospital and have an iron transfusion immediately after the appointment. She expressed her disappointment that this was not arranged for me years earlier. I then realized the seriousness of my situation.

It was at this point I started to feel a little uneasy about what was happening and what was wrong with me. They sat me down on a large recliner in a communal room in the Oncology ward, which was filled with mostly older people receiving their dialysis and chemotherapy treatments. It was a sea of pink-colored gowns and grey hair, along with the moans and groans of tired lungs and joints.

I slunk down in my chair, resting my head on my hand thinking, What the hell am I in for? What's wrong with me? Please tell me I don't have cancer.

Shortly after, a nurse wheeled out the IV machine and what looked like a 2-liter bag[3] filled with a black shimmering, metallic-looking sludge. I went white at the sight of it, and I think at this point I really was on the verge of crapping my pants. It looked so unnatural. In an instant, my 'crapping pants moment' was broken when a hunched over, dear old lady waddled beside me, leaned down, tapped me on the shoulder and said, *"There, there dear, you're going to a better place soon!"*

WHAT THE...? I immediately spluttered with a chuckle and a cry at the same time!

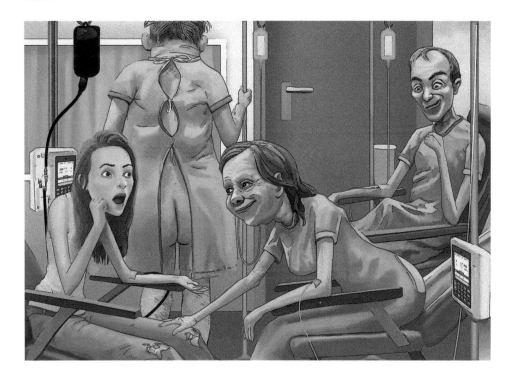

---

[3] Approximately one-half gallon

After the black bag of iron-goop saga finished, I went back to the hematologist. She advised me to get some further blood tests for digestive diseases that could be the cause of my problem. This was news to me. Digestive diseases? I had heard about them, but what did that have to do with me? There was nothing wrong with my digestion. I didn't get sick from food!

She also sent me to have an endoscopy and colonoscopy to check for internal bleeding that could also be a cause. This was going to be a process of elimination, but I wanted to get to the *bottom* of it.

For those of you who do not know what an endoscopy and colonoscopy are, let me have some fun explaining. You go to the hospital, dress up in a tablecloth, and get examined in a manner you'd prefer to avoid. Once you are dazed enough, laying on your side on an examination table with your bare butt exposed to the surgeon and a few other nurses, what comes next is the camera and they have a good snoop around.

So, that's the colonoscopy part, but I had the endoscopy performed at the same time. While I've got my bare ass shining bright like a diamond for all to see, I'm also biting down on a big O-ring that looks a little creepy as they put a camera and some scissors down my throat. It's at this point they took a snippet out of my intestines. This procedure was a first for me and I wished I had been more prepared. If I had known I would be that exposed, I would have freshened up my Brazilian!

A week later, my husband and I were back in the hematologist's office where she delivered the life-changing news…

"You have celiac disease."

What the…? I have celiac disease? I thought to myself.

It felt like I had just been slapped across the face.

My heart sank and in an instant I felt that my life of food, travel, and exploration was over.

So *this* was why I was anemic!

I never knew celiac disease caused vitamin deficiencies. To be honest, I really didn't know much about celiac disease at all except I'd heard people whinge and whine they felt sick, bloated, and couldn't do a poo for a week after eating certain foods.

So, how did she diagnose this precisely?

When I had the scopes done, they took biopsies of my intestinal wall and studied these tissue samples under a microscope and revealed '*100% atrophy of the villi.*' I didn't know what *villi* were, but I knew what *atrophy* meant and it didn't sound good. But what did that mean for me? The hematologist drew a squiggly line on my test results and said, *"This is supposed to be the lining of your intestines; the villi absorb nutrients."* Then she drew a flat line and said, *"You are a flat line."*

The reason my iron was so low was because my guts were essentially **destroyed**, for lack of a better word. I was incapable of absorbing nutrients from my food because I had no villi left. The physical biopsy result, coupled with a blood test for celiac disease, guaranteed an indisputable diagnosis.

She leaned toward me and politely yet sternly said, "From this day forward, **you must never eat gluten again!**"

I looked at her with a blank expression on my face, drew in a deep breath, held back the tears and chirped out, *"What about if I just get IV vitamin transfusions regularly so I can still eat what I want?"*

Typical me, not wanting to take *no* for an answer.

Her response slapped me right in the face, again. "If you continue to eat the way you do now, Jodie, you will end up with a chronic disease very soon. There is too much inflammation going on."

Chronic disease!

Inflammation!

"Basically, Jodie, you're at a much higher risk of developing cancer, and in particular lymphoma cancer, if you keep eating gluten."

In those few moments, I came to the realization that my food would kill me if I didn't change what I ate. Maybe not right now but in time.

I was a healthy, mostly fit, young person who'd just turned 30. I didn't drink fizzy drinks, hardly ever ate chips or bad food except for cheat days, and I took care of myself. So, how and why did I get celiac disease? Why me? Questions flooded my mind. In those moments, in that office, I realized my life was going to change and I wasn't happy about it one little bit.

I went home stunned, still feeling disbelief and trying to register what this really meant for me. It felt so surreal, so unreal, and I felt unsure about the direction my life would take now.

For the first couple of days, I tried to embrace it like a novelty and challenge, similar to the other diet challenges I used to take. However, the heaviness and reality of it all started to set in when I went to reach for some teriyaki sauce to use on my chicken and realized I couldn't have it. This wasn't some novelty diet I could jump in and out of; this would be my life from now on.

Some people make this transition easily and, perhaps for people who have been sick for so long, a diagnosis like this was a blessing. But not for me. It felt like a life sentence. After all, food didn't make me feel sick, so I had no reason to avoid any of it.

"Hey, there are heaps of gluten-free alternatives out there."

And you're right, there are. But what you might not know is that many of those foods can keep you sick and cause further problems down the road. Navigating the ingredients in those products can be a challenge and I'll explain this in later chapters.

As my hematologist said, from that day onward, I wasn't allowed to eat gluten again. So, I didn't.

I went cold turkey, then and there. There was no sneaking one last piece of bread or having a farewell meal (although sometimes I wished I had). I didn't wean myself off gluten like some people might. In part, this was because I was fearful of the big *cancer* word. Also, what if I didn't have enough willpower to kick it fully? What if one last meal turned into one *more* last meal? Either way, I thought it was better to just rip the band-aid off!

During those first couple of days during my cold turkey approach, I ate only fruit, vegetables, and meat while I contemplated an action plan.

Job Number 1: I had to do my research on what exactly gluten *was* and in what food products it was found. I knew the usual products like bread and pasta, but I had no idea just how complex this ingredient was and how widely it was used in other food products.

Job Number 2: Clean out the fridge and cupboards.

I grabbed a large heavy-duty plastic garbage bag, rolled up my sleeves, put on rubber gloves, and wore my husband's safety goggles. I turned up the stereo and conveniently enough Bob Marley bellowed through the speakers.

"Don't worry, about a thing. 'Cause every little thing's gonna be alright."

I rummaged through my pantry and tossed out some of my most valued possessions. My angel hair pasta that I used to make with fresh chili, garlic, and crab. **Gone!**

My instant pepper Gravox mix that I used on a rosemary seasoned lamb rack. **Gone!** *(Don't make fun of my instant gravy, it was the best!)*

The list went on and my bags were filling up.

Hours later, I was sitting on the floor in front of the fridge with a pile of condiments around me that I could no longer eat. Don't even get me started on the traditional prawn gyoza I had in the freezer. *Ohh nooo,* I thought. *My Aussie meat pies.* They're a time-honored tradition in Australia. This can't possibly get any worse. Oh, but it did.

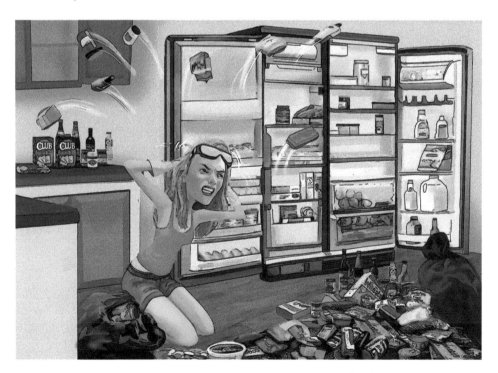

If anyone had seen me, they would have thought, *She's lost her bloody mind; it's just gluten.* In all honesty, I think I did lose my mind when I saw how many products contain gluten. There it was, the word **gluten** sticking out like dog's balls on my favorite food products.

No more crumbed barramundi fish and beer battered chips. No more sushi rolls. No more burritos. And beer. Are you serious? What was I going to drink after a day of working hard in the garden? What about when I sat down with my cowboy/farmer dad and couldn't have a beer with him anymore? Not the beer!

Days turned into weeks, weeks turned into months, and I was still struggling. I hardly ever went out to eat. I was too embarrassed and got upset every time I saw delicious-looking food I couldn't have.

Eating out with my husband was a major part of our life and a significant part of my life as a foodie. I wasn't one of those people who analyzed the menus and had to ask, *"What's in that?"* or *"Do you have anything gluten-free?"* So, the thought of doing this made me churn with embarrassment and shame. I felt like I was missing out on life and now *I* was becoming *the difficult one* at a restaurant.

On the odd couple of occasions we went out during this time, the difficult nature of this diagnosis was reinforced. At one cafe, the menu was unclear and the waitress unhelpful, so I ordered a poached egg, a piece of tomato, and a bit of avocado. Plain and downright boring.

One of the worst situations was when my husband and I went to a place we frequented before my diagnosis and asked if they had anything gluten-free. The young girl behind the counter went to the kitchen to ask the chef, and moments later the chef came out in haste with a somewhat annoyed look upon her face. She blurted, *"Are you celiac or just gluten-free?"*

I replied, *"I'm Celiac,"* and before I could say any more, she snapped back at me with, *"I can't cook for your kind here."*

I was stunned and shocked. All sorts of things were going through my head at that moment, mostly because I didn't know whether I was going to cry or crawl over the countertop and whack her across the face with a baguette for being so mean to me. She obviously saw the thoughts running through my mind and quickly backed herself up saying, *"My kitchen is not equipped to cook for celiacs!"* and darted away out of sight.

The fact that my first few dining out experiences were terrible only made things worse.

I was beginning to feel depressed and quite sorry for myself. I'd always been one to keep my emotions away from friends and family, but I found myself telling anyone who would listen about my *horrific* (as I thought of it) story. I guess I wanted sympathy but mostly all I received from people was, *"It's not that bad," "There's plenty of options out there," "Everyone caters for gluten-intolerant people nowadays,"* and the comments went on.

None of them made me feel any better; if anything, I felt worse because I felt like my emotions and what I was going through were being dismissed. I really felt like no one could understand what it meant for me and the changes and sacrifices I had to consciously make. I didn't know of anyone else with celiac disease that I could talk to, so I was on my own in this.

I'd eaten my way around many countries in the world, and I worried about how limited my culinary adventures would be in the future. How hard would it be when I traveled? Was I now going to be that *high maintenance* girl? You know, the one who says, *"Oh what's in that?"* or *"I can't have that?"* or *"Do you have anything gluten-free?"* I couldn't ever stand those types of people, and now I was one of them.

Then the tears started again. *Geez, I'm crying a lot lately. This is so not me*, I thought to myself. Several times over that period, I felt myself tear up, including when I went to the latest food and wine show. There I was, no longer able to pick at the sample trays people were holding out trying to tantalize my taste buds. I looked around and realized I was limited to about 20% of the food there. Again, my heart sank. Why did I even bother to go?

Since I'd cut out gluten, I felt like my body was falling apart. The skin on my face was so itchy I wanted to claw it off any chance I got. The dermatitis I had when I was a child seemed to have come back and the moods, boy did I have some seriously massive mood swings. My nasal passages clogged up so bad I thought I had a cold for months. But I wasn't sick with the flu. Sometimes I didn't know if I was coming or going or happy or sad. I felt like I was having one of those menstrual cycle mood swings but amplified by 100. If you're a female reading this book, you know just how out-of-mind you can feel and if you're a guy reading this book, I'm sure you have had a girlfriend or wife who turned into something that reminded you of the crazy ugly demon from the movie *The Exorcist!*

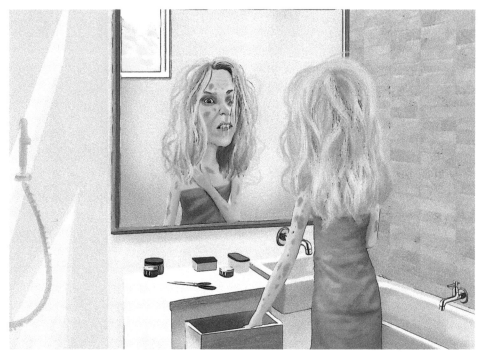

What the hell was going on? I'd never had any problems when I ate gluten-containing foods and now since cutting it out, I seemed to have a whole basket full of problems. This seriously could not get any worse. Tie a brick to my feet and chuck me in the deep end, I thought!

I finally and reluctantly went to Dr. Google, read forum after forum and found out that, for some people, gluten can act like a drug and going cold turkey can cause withdrawal symptoms. I thought, *Ha, you really know how to do a number on yourself don't you? This just gets better and better.* It seemed other people on the forums complained of the same concerns as mine, plus more, for either weeks or months at a time. Who would have thought withdrawal symptoms could last for so bloody long and you could get it from food? I didn't know if this thought enraged me for these poor sufferers or comforted me knowing I was not alone. I did some research and it turned out that wheat can have the same addictive hold over the brain as opium! Was I getting high off my bread?

I looked like crap, I felt like crap, and my life was now crap. I was feeling more and more depressed, and finally the stress of it all got to me.

This is it—major meltdown time!

My husband was away working overseas and we were talking on the phone. I burst into tears telling him how sick I was and how much I was struggling. I thought I was losing my mind.

He had such patience about this whole situation and he couldn't have conducted himself better, actually. He wanted to eat everything I had to eat, he never complained, and always tried to make me feel like it wasn't that big of a deal, that I could get through this.

But that night I poured a glass of wine—well, it was more like the size of a medieval goblet—and I wailed like a spoiled brat who wasn't getting what she wanted. I just let loose on the poor guy expecting sympathy and understanding from him.

When he'd had enough of my ranting and raving, his nurturing on that call turned into tough love. It most certainly wasn't what I was expecting nor wanting. I was hoping for sympathy, empathy, and for him to console me again like all the other times. But what I received instead was the biggest kick up the ass!

"Jodie, you're better than this," he said. "You have gone vegan, paleo, neolithic, every type of diet known to man, experimenting for fun and you dragged me along with you. You know the reason why you need to have this new way of life. If the case was reversed and I was diagnosed, you would have changed your way of life in an instant without a blink of an eye…for me! Yet you can't seem to do it for yourself. Why can't you just deal with this? Enough is enough, Jodie!"

I gasped in horror at the unexpected blasting I received, chugged down my glass of wine, and let the tears roll.

He was so right. Why was this so hard for me? Not hearing a response from me (first time in a long time again; I was silent for a change) he continued, "Just think about the poor people who go into anaphylactic shock after trace amounts of nuts. That will kill them in an instant; this will not! And the real reason you're struggling to deal with this is that little Miss Jodie doesn't have a choice in the matter. You're not in control anymore and that scares the hell out of you."

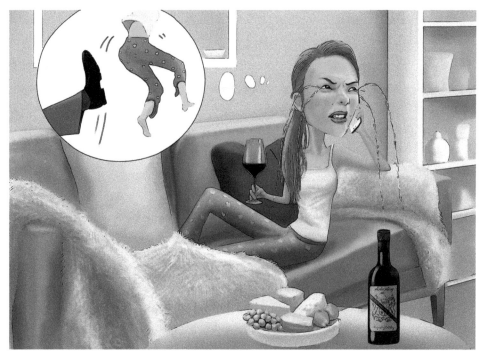

There it was. All the honesty cards on the table. Why couldn't I come to understand this earlier? Who knows, maybe I did, but I didn't want to believe it. After an hour's conversation and getting this long overdue kick up the butt, we said our goodnights. As I slid further into the couch, clutching my vintage Shiraz in one hand and my smoked cheese in the other, I *reflected*.

Oddly enough, I woke the next morning with some miraculous new-found freedom *and* a headache. *Surprise, surprise!* I felt free of the guilt, shame, and self-pity. I needed to take back control. I guess the previous night's kick up the butt really got through to me, or the Shiraz was a bottle of magical mojo.

For the first time since my diagnosis, I actually felt like I could embrace my new path. I had no choice really and now I knew that. *Who knows? With my geekiness for research and health maybe I could write a book one day?* I thought.

After going cold turkey, I would say it took around four months of emotional and physical torture before I felt better and felt myself again. Once I got over the unexpected detoxing from gluten:

- my waistline seemed to be a little flatter and less bloated,

- my energy levels seemed to pick up, and

- I was no longer blowing my nose every day with the feeling of having a mysterious flu.

Not only did my current suffering symptoms ease, but other ailments I'd lived with and considered normal started to get better too. The dark circles I'd had under my eyes for as long as I could remember seemed to disappear! I had recently burned my arm with hot oil while cooking and had a big bright red blister mark. Usually, whenever I was hurt, cut, or scraped it could take over six months for the wound to heal. I thought that was normal. But after 10 days my burn had healed completely.

Overall, I was feeling more comfortable in my skin. It was almost like things started to function better, perhaps as they should have. It's a bizarre feeling to describe, but I started to feel amazing.

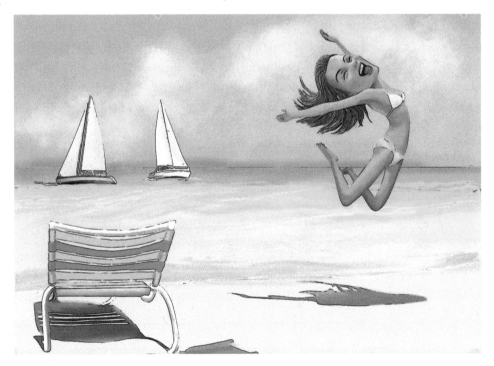

I spent the next few years researching gluten, inflammation, and people's reactions to both. I wanted to know all about it. I wanted to know the hows, the whys, and all the in-betweens.

I found tons of books saying the typical *avoid gluten* to fix the problem, and I found some people's books on how easy it was for them to transition to a GF lifestyle. I also found a lot of stories like mine. Well, worse actually, which made me realize that others really had it tough for a long time and a diagnosis was a blessing not a curse.

However, there were only a few books that combined the gluten-free lifestyle and information on inflammation. Inflammation is a key point that not many people understand.

This is where my book comes into play.

As I said at the beginning of the book, what once was a terrible diagnosis became my new adventure in life. I want to supercharge you with knowledge about gluten, celiac disease, and especially inflammation and how it impacts the body. Sometimes, if we have a better understanding for the whats and whys, the hows become much easier.

I want to show you how to transition to a gluten-free lifestyle much more effortlessly than I did and give you a tool chest of resources for understanding your disease better, tips on how to heal your body faster, guides for dining out, traveling, and what your emergency kit might be for those unsuspected gluten invasion moments. I want to hold your hand through this period and to hopefully inspire you with new information on how to live a long, happy, and healthy gluten-free life.

This book is my gift to you.

Chapter 3

Digestion *101*

*B*efore we jump into the nuts and bolts of celiac disease, it will all make more sense if we have a better understanding of what happens to the body when we eat food, especially considering that celiac disease is a digestive disease!

I was chatting with the lady who does my nails about celiac disease and she explained she had just been diagnosed with type 2 diabetes. She was quite confused about the whole thing and didn't understand what the doctors were saying. I wasn't surprised in the least to hear that.

Wanting to show off my geeky (un-doctored) knowledge of the body, I broke it down to her in very simple terms, with some fun analogies about what diabetes is, probable causes, and what's happening to her body every time she eats or drinks something. She looked at me and said, *"Thank you. No one has ever explained it to me like that before. I knew nothing about the digestive system or how the body works. That makes much more sense now."*

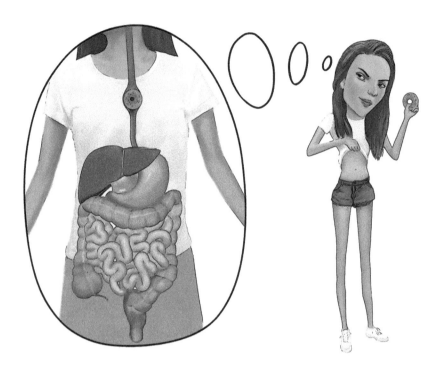

It was at this point that I realized not too many people know how the digestive system works. Truth be told, I was no expert either and only gained a more in-depth knowledge after my celiac diagnosis. Celiac disease is a disorder to the digestive system caused by eating gluten. I wanted to learn all about how the digestive process works so I could take back some control in this matter. I felt like the more I knew, the more tools I had to deal with this disease, understand any issues, and overcome adverse situations. This was my body and something's gone haywire, so the more I know about it, the better I can manage it through life. For some, learning about this type of information can be as boring as watching grass grow, but when you think about it, it's quite an integral thing to understand, especially when you have a digestive disorder. So, I've done the hard work for you by extracting information from multiple sources and, hopefully, my creative little descriptions of your pipework are good enough for you to enjoy and learn from.

So, if you have little knowledge of the inner workings of your pipes, before skipping to the next chapter, have a read below.

I don't remember where I heard or read it, but this little saying has stayed with me constantly: **the digestive tract that runs through the body is the only thing that connects us with the outside world.**

Your organs are completely protected from the elements of the outside world. Our skin is a barrier; our eyes, nails and hair all protect us so the bad stuff can't get in.

So, it would make sense that the tube that runs from your mouth, down through the center of your body, right to your anus *is* what connects the inside of us to the world around us. That tube is about 30 feet long, or 30 packets of spaghetti joined together. In my case, it's five times the length of my entire body! If that's still hard to imagine, then picture a three-story building. It's strange to think that such a mega long tube is crumpled up inside my belly.

This tube is called a *musculo-membranous* tube, meaning it is both muscle and membrane. Another similar description of a muscle-membrane tube is the vagina, and I'm sure nearly everyone reading this book, male or female, knows what a vagina feels like.

Did you know that the very first part of a baby that develops in the womb is actually the anus[4]? Yes, that's right. We all started our life out as assholes. Literally!

The anus cells develop first, followed by nerve cells, which then begin to form the first of your vital organs. From this, your digestive tract is one of the very first parts of you that develops. Your digestive tract is how you interact with the world, yet it remains one of the least known parts of the body.

If I asked you what your heart, lungs, and liver do, I'm sure you would have answers like:

- A muscle that pumps blood
- Air sacs that allow me to breathe
- An organ that filters my blood

But what if I asked you what your bowel is responsible for? Or what does your stomach do? Most people would respond with, "Bowel is for pooping and stomach

---

[4] Keeton, W. and Sircus, W. (2016). "Invertebrate digestive system." Encyclopaedia Britannica. Retrieved from: https://www.britannica.com/science/human-digestive-system/The-gastrointestinal-tract-as-an-organ-of-immunity#ref294250

is to digest food." While this is correct to a very—and only very—slight degree, most of us *don't* really know what's going on inside the body that we live with for decades upon decades.

How many times have you eaten something, become bloated, and clutched the area below your belly button saying, *"I feel sick in my stomach?"* Would it surprise you to know that what you're clutching is your small intestine, which is what's probably giving you grief, and not your stomach? Your stomach is actually located under the last five ribs on the left-hand side of your body. Put your left hand underneath your left breast (for both male and female) and line up your fingertips to the center of your body. That's where your stomach is and you should feel the bottom of your rib cage with the side edge of your palm. The size of your hand and where you're touching right now is almost the size and location of your stomach!

To help you understand the different areas and functions along the 30 feet of pipework, I've made a quick organ description to start, then a creative break down from start to finish, or '*mouth to bum hole!*'

1. **The Mouth (The Masticator)** – Process of chewing food and the role of saliva.

2. **The Pharynx (The Throat)** – Understanding the importance of food going down the right tube.

3. **The Esophagus (The Gullet)** – The start of your unconsciously controlled muscles.

4. **The Stomach (The Acrobatic Washing Machine)** – Acids, washing machine suds, alcohol, and medications.

5. **The Small Intestine (The Magic Maker)** – The life or death of your nutrient-capturing sea anemone.

6. **The Large Intestine (The Poop Shoot)** – The fermentation tube that's home to trillions of bacteria responsible for your survival.

The mouth (the masticator)

Hmm, I like the sound of that word…*masticator*. It sounds like some medieval torture method. Oxford dictionary describes the word *masticator* as '*a machine for grinding or pulping material*' and that's exactly what it does. It grinds your food.

When you bite down into a hot fresh cinnamon doughnut, the first thing you do is chew. This is the very beginning of the digestive process and what better way to start than with some of the strongest muscles in your body: the jaw muscles and tongue.

When you bite, you can exert up to approximately 75kg (171 pounds) of pressure for molar teeth[5]. That's more than my own body weight! So perhaps the saying *'you could chew your own arm off'* might actually be real. If you haven't heard of that saying before…if you've ever had a drunken night out on the town and hooked up with a guy or a girl then woken up the next morning to realize they look nothing like you thought, you would rather chew your own arm off and sneak out before waking them up. *(I got the strangest look from my husband when he read this part of the book.)*

Anyway, back to that doughnut in your mouth. You're chomping, chewing, and grinding, but we need something else to water it down and that is *saliva*.

Saliva is produced from a few different glands around your mouth. They are under your tongue, by your jawline, and in front of your ear. The gland near your ear squirts saliva into your mouth and onto your tongue through a tube in either side of your cheek like a little water gun whenever you put something in your mouth.

The glands under your tongue produce saliva all day long like a broken record, and they don't produce just a little. It's a lot. Upwards to nearly a liter[6] a day.

The human body is such an amazing thing that it can even produce saliva by thought, hence the term *mouth-watering*. I'm sure at one point in your life you've seen a gooey, rich piece of cake and suddenly it feels like your mouth is literally filling up with saliva. That's your body pre-empting what's about to happen and kickstarting your digestive process in anticipation. This process is controlled by the nervous system that runs right through your body and connects your gut to your brain. You *see* a piece of cake, *think* how delicious it would be, and your nerves signal your gut to get prepared for a deluge of cake.

I don't even have to see food to start the waterworks; I can just imagine it. I can imagine a lemon—the skin, the color, and the sharp sour taste—then before I

---

[5] "The Power of the Human Jaw". (1911). *Scientific American, 105(*23*)*, 493.
doi:10.1038/scientificamerican12021911-493
[6] About 2 pints

can feel my saliva glands activate. It's the strangest sensation. Talk about
matter!

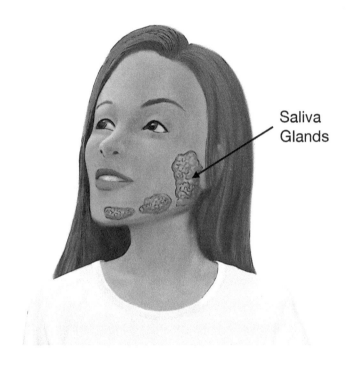

Saliva
Glands

That clear, slimy goop that forms in your mouth is mostly water and made
from filtered blood. However, it also contains electrolytes, mucus, antibacterial
compounds, and other various enzymes. It can tell us so much about the body. It
is used in DNA mapping and can also be tested for diseases.

One other really cool thing about saliva is that it contains a painkiller stronger
than morphine[7]! Even though we try to chew our food to a paste, sometimes we
don't always do a good job. Can you imagine how much more uncomfortable it
would be if we swallowed the chunky food down without any of that magic
painkiller in our saliva? Ever had a corn chip scrape down your throat? Without
some painkiller-containing saliva, it could hurt like hell.

Have you ever heard someone say, *"The mouth is the fastest healing part of
the whole body?"* Well, they're right, along with the cornea in the eye. Do you

---

[7] Wisner, A., Dufour, E., Messaoudi, M., Nejdi, A., Marcel, A., Ungeheuer, M., Rougeot, C.
(2006). "Human Opiorphin, a natural antinociceptive modulator of opioid-dependent pathways."
Proceedings of the National Academy of Sciences, Nov. 2006, *103*(47) 17979-17984.
doi:10.1073/pnas.0605865103

remember when you burned your mouth eating something hot, or you chomped down hard on the side of your mouth and pierced your cheek, only to find a few hours later that it's already healing over? Well, you can thank your saliva for that. Its healing and antibacterial properties are off the charts. It's not only good for healing the mouth, but it's also good for helping to kill the bacteria in your food so you don't get sick.

Chewing your food properly is *so* important; I can't stress that enough. The more you chew, the more saliva you produce with all those amazing benefits, which means the food is more digestible and less work for your stomach.

Savor the flavor of your food and help kick start the process for your digestive system by chewing more so your guts don't have to work so hard. This chewing part of the digestive process is the only part over which you have conscious control. Once you swallow the food, that's it; your body's automation takes over.

The pharynx (the throat)

Once you've chewed your food and swallowed, the food is pushed to the back of the mouth by your tongue to the *throat,* technically called the *pharynx.* This tube is about 4 inches long and connects from the nasal cavity at the back of your mouth to the top of the esophagus about halfway down your neck, roughly behind the Adam's Apple on a man.

When you swallow, breathing has to stop. The muscles at the top of the throat behind the mouth shut off access to the nasal pipes going up, and a special flap at the bottom of the throat snaps shut over the opening of the windpipe to make sure the food is diverted down the right pipe.

Sitting directly in front of your *throat/pharynx* is your *windpipe,* technically called the *trachea.* The trachea is where air flows in and out of your lungs. These two pipes, your *throat* and *windpipe,* sit one in front of the other and look like one tube split in half.

Sometimes when you're really distracted, or doing too many things at once like chomping down on your toast and slurping your coffee while yelling at the kids to get ready for school and packing their lunches *(take a breath),* your brain misfires and forgets to shut the flap in time and the food accidentally goes down your windpipe. In a fraction of a second, little nerves inside your windpipe have sensed the food and immediately make you cough and splutter the food back up.

You will either cough it up and out your mouth, or it bounces into your throat and down your esophagus.

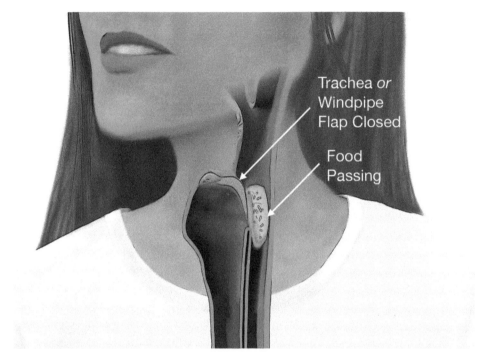

Trachea *or* Windpipe Flap Closed

Food Passing

I've seen this first-hand when I joked to my mother on April Fool's Day that I was pregnant while she was taking a sip of wine. Not only did she seem to choke, she involuntarily spat the wine right out of her mouth in a split second! I would definitely assume something distracted her a little too much.

Once the food has properly entered the throat, the muscles inside contract, pushing the food down and into your esophagus.

The esophagus (the gullet)

When I think of an esophagus, oddly enough, I imagine a pelican's neck. The esophagus is about nine inches long and connects from the base of the pharynx (roughly the midline of your neck) down to the stomach pouch. The top third of the esophagus is lined with a special muscle that allows you to feel the food moving through. However, that muscle changes around the location of your breastbone and you can no longer feel the food traveling anymore. I'm sure that, at least once in your lifetime, on a boiling day, you've felt icy cold water slide down your throat but then disappear somewhere around your chest area.

The muscle lining of the esophagus works to push food down like a Mexican wave at a concert...*or* think of a snake eating a mouse. The tube constricts behind the food, pushing it along while the lower part opens up to receive it, then constricts again behind it, eventually pushing the food all the way to the stomach pouch opening. The lining of the esophagus squirts out another type of mucus to help lubricate the food on its way down and has a special membrane lining to protect it from damage. It has to withstand abrasive food fragments like fish bones, rough fibrous vegetables, *and* Doritos®, so we really don't want there to be any punctures along the way. The esophagus does not absorb nutrients; its job is to simply pass the food from the mouth to the stomach.

The timing for solid foods to get from your mouth to the opening of your stomach is up to eight seconds. For liquids it's much quicker, around two to three seconds.

At the base of your esophagus and the start of the stomach is a sphincter, much like the one in your bum. When you swallow food, this sphincter, along with the flap at the top of your esophagus, shuts close to prevent air from getting into the digestive tract. Heartburn, reflux, and even burping occurs when the lower sphincter does not close properly.

The body is designed to let excess gases and air out of the digestive tract with burping and farting. This is an involuntary action that not too many people have control over, so the next time your friend burps the alphabet at the dinner table thinking it's funny, congratulate them on their talent and ability to control their sphincter.

Aside from keeping air out, this sphincter valve has another job: to keep food down in your stomach and not let it go back up again. However, if you've ever eaten something terrible, like an *off* prawn at a dodgy restaurant, you may have vomited. In that instance, the entire system of what I've just described works in the reverse.

The sphincter valve opens up and those Mexican-hat-wave muscles pump the food from the stomach up and back out the mouth, sometimes *so* quickly that you don't even know it's happening until it's too late.

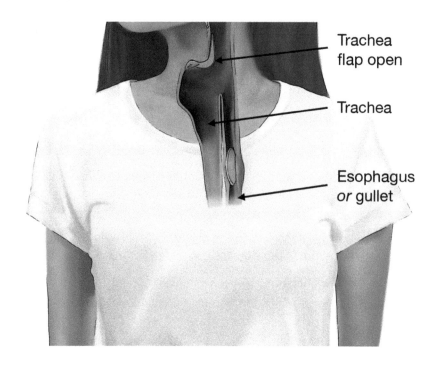

Trachea
flap open

Trachea

Esophagus
or gullet

That, my dear friends, is what's called vomiting, and it's your body's way of saying to whatever the hell was in there, *"Get the hell out!"*

The ugly part of vomiting is that you might feel a burning acidic sensation in your throat or mouth. That is stomach acid and guess what the main ingredient is? Hydrochloric acid! Have you ever vomited so much that there is nothing left, but you kept vomiting and got a clear, yellow-tinted glue-like substance? That is bile. Yuck.

The stomach (the acrobatic washing machine)

Your stomach is located on your left-hand side of your body, half underneath your rib cage and tucked in behind the liver. I call the stomach a *pouch* as it looks like the pouch on a set of Scottish bagpipes, but it's still part of the same tube from your mouth to your butt. It's just a different shape, has different muscles, and is up to 12 inches long. The connection point of the esophagus to the stomach pouch is off to one side rather than straight down from the top. This is a particularly good design to keep food moving through the system and not just bouncing back up whenever it can. The stomach is pliable, stretches like pizza dough, and relaxes like a chilled-out Rastafarian when food gets shoved in from the sphincter at the base of the esophagus. The process is similar to shoving someone through a door and slamming it shut behind them. The stomach is so relaxed and stretchy that you can easily fit an entire loaf of bread into it if you wanted to. *(Warning: please do not try this at home.)*

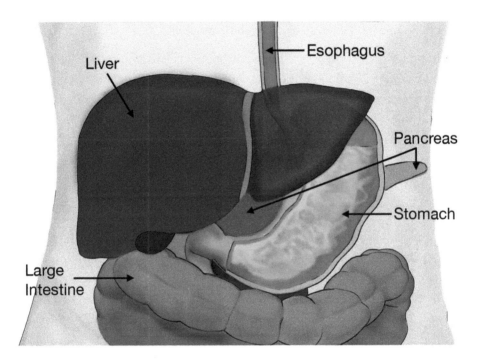

Once your food has reached the stomach, the acrobatic washing machine switches on. The walls of your stomach begin to smash and pummel the food from one side to another. Think of your dirty clothes tumbling in the washer time and time again in the churning water. Now the washing machine suds are activated. Your stomach spurts out enzymes, to help break down proteins, and detergents in the form of bile to help breakdown fats. Could you imagine how coagulated fat would get in your gut if it didn't have some soap suds to help? Among the enzymes and suds is also acid, which helps to kill off bacteria that might lurk in the food. This acid also reduces the pH level of the contents in your guts.

This process can take up to two hours for fruits and vegetables, and for meats it can be somewhere up to six hours to complete. However, simple carbohydrates (like pasta, bread, and cake) can make it pretty quickly into the *small intestine*, the next part of the digestive system, in record time: under 30 minutes.

The stomach, being pliable, can expand to two liters[8] in size. That's massive! To put that in perspective, hold a two-liter container of milk or soda across the middle of your stomach and see how big it is. For me it covers the entire breadth of my midsection, yet all my other organs are in there too. No wonder I feel like a pregnant lady after eating at a buffet. It pushes my other poor organs out of the way while I bloat outward; I've stretched it to the limit! Thinking about it like that now, I don't think I'll ever go back to a buffet again!

Your gut is pretty good at telling your brain when to stop eating. On average, it can take around 20 minutes of eating for the stomach to signal the brain that it's full and to stop shoving more food in. Therefore, when you take time chewing your food, you won't be able to eat as much food as you normally could. Weight-loss tip: chew your food for longer so you don't eat as much!

Even though the stomach can expand to two liters in size, you can still shovel more food down your gullet if you want to. You only have to look at those eating contests where the guy or girl eats 15 burgers in one session.

To combat your horrible and punishing attitude toward your body, the stomach has a fail-safe. It's very well connected to the nervous system. If you overeat more than your stomach can handle, it signals to the muscles of your gut to increase the speed with which it needs to push food through the rest of the digestive system. So, rather than allowing your stomach to do its job well, it opens the floodgates and off goes the food into your intestines before it's ready. Then your intestines open their flood gates and push the food out. Ever seen someone at a buffet go off to the toilet for a poo, only to come back to eat more food now that they've made room?

The stomach also does not absorb much at all in the way of nutrients, but what it absorbs is water, along with other molecules such as medications, caffeine, and alcohol. The lining of the stomach is not as tough as the lining of the esophagus and can be damaged quite easily by chemicals. That's why we are told to eat food when taking some medications.

Once the body senses that the food particles are broken down to about the size of two millimeters (less than half a grain of rice) the next sphincter door, located at the bottom of the stomach and at the entry to the small intestine, opens and shuts.

---

[8] About a half-gallon

Again, the shoving of the food from the stomach to the small intestine occurs with the slamming of the door behind it.

The food passed into the small intestine is now called *chyme*. The smoothie-like consistency got its name from Greek origins meaning *juice*. So gross! I would not want to vomit that back up, that's for sure! Think of a cheap sausage from the supermarket, the ones where it is all one pinkish color. Now, squeeze the sausage contents out, and that's getting close to what *chyme* is.

The small intestine (the magic maker)

I call the small intestine the magic maker as it's the part of the digestive system responsible for extracting nutrients from the food and sending it to other parts of your body. To me, that's the magic part.

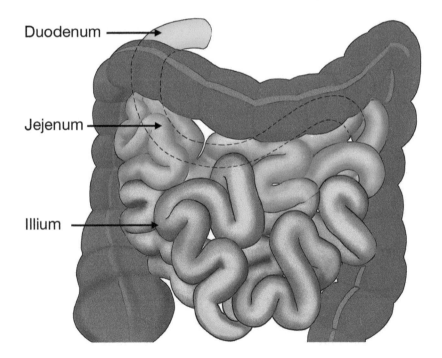

Overall, the small intestine is up to 20 feet long and is broken down into three stages. Each of the three stages has a unique role in the digestion and absorption of nutrients from food.

- Stage 1 - the duodenum
- Stage 2 - the jejunum

- Stage 3 - the ilium

There *are* small amounts of bacteria in your small intestine; however, most of the bacteria your digestive system carries are in your large intestine. Food can take between one to four hours for processing in the small intestine, depending on what you've eaten.

On the inside, the chyme is pushed through the small intestine in a corkscrew fashion, winding its way through 20 feet of tube. If you were to look at it from the outside, the small intestine still moves like a Mexican wave, but because of the unique contour of the intestine, your chyme corkscrews its way through. If there wasn't a special layer of fat and muscle between your intestines and your skin, you would be able to feel the whole process if you put your hand on your belly!

Stage 1 - the duodenum

Once the chyme is pushed through the sphincter valve at the end of the stomach, it enters the *duodenum.* The duodenum is a short section at the start of the small intestine approximately 30 centimeters[9] long.

When the chyme leaves the stomach it has a pH rating of around 2. Would you believe that's only slightly higher than the acid levels of a dog's stomach (pH approx. 1.5)? That's amazing considering dogs can break down solid bones in their stomachs. Before you think about eating bones, the answer is *no.* We can't eat bones like dogs do.

Once the duodenum feels the food inside, it secretes a hormone that activates the gallbladder to release an alkaline bile into the mix. That same hormone also activates the *pancreas* to secrete digestive enzymes and bicarbonate soda. The digestive enzymes, along with the alkaline bile and bi-carb soda, work together to raise the pH level back up to around 7, so the food is at a safe level to move throughout the small intestine. We wouldn't want our delicate intestines to be burned from all that acid now, would we?

Stage 2 - the jejunum

Once the food has its pH balance restored, it then moves into the second stage of the intestine called the *jejunum.* This second stage of the small intestine is three

---

[9] Approximately 12 inches

to six feet long and is responsible for the absorption of proteins, carbohydrates, amino acids, sugar, fatty acids, fat-soluble vitamins (A, D, & E), minerals, electrolytes, and water.

Stage 3 – the ileum

The ileum is about another 6-12 feet long before it attaches to the *large intestine,* aka the *poop shoot*! It mainly absorbs vitamin B12 and other water-soluble vitamins (B-group, folate, biotin, pantothenic acid, vitamin C), bile, salts, and other nutrients that were not absorbed in Stage 2.

Overall

The inside walls of your 20-foot-long small intestinal tube is lined with *heaps* of tissue folds, kind of like a Shar Pei dog, or a rolly polly, as I like to call them. The idea behind these folds of tissues is to increase the surface area that can come in contact with the chyme.

Drill down even further microscopically and you find that these tissue folds are covered in hairy-like fingers (called villi) that sway back and forth like a sea anemone, and these too increase the surface area again. In one square inch of tissue there is up to 20,000 villi. Drill down even further microscopically, and each of those 20,000 villi have their own set of miniature villi attached to them called microvilli. This equates to around 130 billion microvilli per square inch.

The villi that line the entire of the small intestine are at their longest inside stage 2. If you laid all your villi out flat, they would nearly cover the size of a tennis court. These hairy-like structures catch the nutrients from food as it passes through the intestines, much like a sea anemone catches microscopic nutrients from the surrounding seawater.

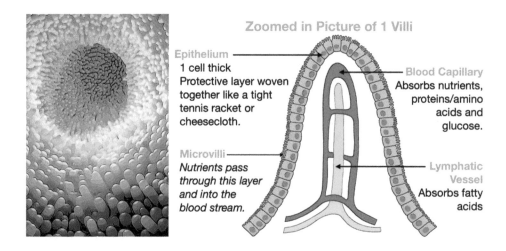

Zoomed in Picture of 1 Villi

Epithelium
1 cell thick
Protective layer woven together like a tight tennis racket or cheesecloth.

Blood Capillary
Absorbs nutrients, proteins/amino acids and glucose.

Microvilli
Nutrients pass through this layer and into the blood stream.

Lymphatic Vessel
Absorbs fatty acids

The villi then pass these nutrients through the lining of the intestinal wall into the bloodstream where they are carried first to the liver to be cleansed of toxins, medication residues, and so on. Then the nutrients are shipped off to various parts of your body. This includes other organs, your brain, your skin—basically everywhere. It spreads nutrients around as fast as a viral post on Facebook!

Your pancreas measures the amount of sugar in your blood. When it senses that the sugar levels are too high, it releases insulin into the blood, which then stores those sugars in your cells, which turns into fat to be used later. Back in caveman days, this design worked perfectly; however, today is a different story. Most of us don't use the fat for energy later and just keep getting fatter.

The insulin levels in your blood should look like the rolling waves of the ocean, but when you eat high carbohydrate foods like bread for breakfast, sandwiches and bagels for lunch, then pasta for dinner, your insulin levels look like jagged mountain peaks and valleys, and don't get a chance to rest. If this keeps up, you can develop insulin resistance. Insulin resistance can then lead to diabetes.

Think back to your first alcoholic drink; it most likely made your legs, arms, and head feel tingly and you felt drunk pretty quickly. Over time, your body adapts so it takes much more alcohol than before to get drunk and give you those same feelings. That's resistance, and the same thing can happen with your insulin.

Have you ever felt *exhausted* when you've eaten too much? That feeling where you want to just flop on the couch, cradle your belly, and can't even decide what to watch on TV? You feel as if you're in a food coma. Well, all that food you just ate requires a large amount of energy and blood to process. The body has this wonderful thing where it can divert close to a third of the body's blood to the digestive tract. That blood is pumped from the less important body parts that are required after a meal, like your arms, legs…even your head! So, now you know why you get that foggy brain feeling after a big meal. My theory is that your arms, legs, and head that would be used in a fight-or-flight situation should not be required after a heavy meal, as there is no perceived threat nearby. It seems to be a very primitive response.

The large intestine (the poop shoot)

Once food has passed through the small intestine, it's ready to enter the *large intestine*, again through another sphincter door. The large intestine measures about five feet long, is twice the width of the small intestine, and is broken down into seven stages:

- Stage 1 - cecum
- Stage 2 - ascending colon
- Stage 3 - transverse colon
- Stage 4 - descending colon
- Stage 5 - sigmoid colon
- Stage 6 - rectum
- Stage 7 - anal canal

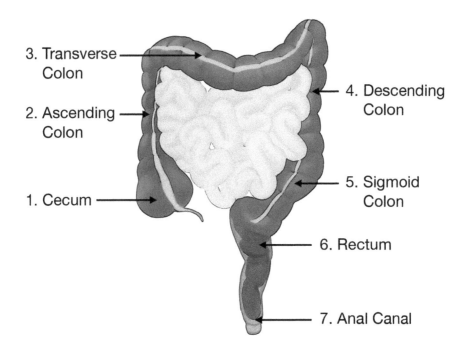

3. Transverse Colon

2. Ascending Colon

1. Cecum

4. Descending Colon

5. Sigmoid Colon

6. Rectum

7. Anal Canal

If you were looking at it on someone else, it would look like a square question mark. When looking at yourself, it starts on the right-hand side of your body inside your hip cavity.

Connecting from your small intestine is a pouch (cecum) that starts about two inches lower than the top of your hip bone and extends all the way vertically (ascending colon) to the underside of the last two ribs. It then goes horizontally across your midsection (transverse colon) and tucks in under the last two ribs on the left-hand side before making its way down inside your left hip (descending colon). It then goes horizontally again backward toward your tailbone (sigmoid colon) before heading downward between your bum cheeks (rectum). Here it is greeted by another sphincter valve to the anal canal, which is approximately 1.5 inches long. At the end of the anal canal is your anus (the beginning of your life, if you remember the start of the chapter) and the end of your digestive tube and the connection back to the outside world.

Even though I tease the large intestine with the name of the *poop shoot*, it's far more than that. It plays a major role in extracting the final nutrients from your food, houses most of the bacteria in your digestive system, plays a major role in the health of your immune system, and it talks to your brain…quite a lot!

There is so much special bacteria in your colon that medical procedures are being developed called fecal transplants. Basically, they transfer the poo and bacteria from one person to help cure disease in another.

The large intestine (the poop shoot) extracts out the last of the nutrients possible from the food. However, there are no villi lining the large intestine; it's just lined with smooth tissue cells that do the job instead. It then also extracts any water it can, turning the leftover food into a more solid material people politely call poo.

Food can last in the large intestine from 18 hours to two days, again depending on what you eat, so you can imagine how old the food is in your large intestine if you're constipated. It could get a little toxic and putrid if it stays in there for too long, and unfortunately, the cell wall may reabsorb some of the putrid bacteria back into your body, so it's vital that we eliminate waste effectively.

Warning: Just like all the valves from your stomach and throat can open to get you to vomit, your intestinal sphincters can also do the same in reverse if you eat something that the body *really* doesn't like. It can have a funny way of activating the uncontrollable release of your faithful internal anal sphincter, putting that much pressure on your bum hole to hold back the sheer force that's pushing on it. Sometimes when it's that bad, there is a fine line we might be forced to cross, so know where the exits are at all times.

Once the food is shoved into your large intestine, it enters the *cecum* (first stage) and is mixed with the first round of bacteria who are comfortably living in this space. The bacteria living in this chamber can be quite old and have probably been living and growing with you throughout your lifetime. Bacteria live throughout your large intestine, but it's this chamber that seems to store the oldest bacteria, simply because the chamber drops down into a sac.

Once the food has been formally introduced to round one of bacteria, it is then pumped upward through the *ascending colon* then through the rest of your large intestine. While the food passes through the rest of the intestine, it undergoes a bacterial fermentation process to release more water-soluble vitamins for absorption that could not be done in the small intestine.

The colon bacteria are almost solely responsible for producing vitamin K, which is vital for blood clotting, and the absorption of calcium. As mentioned before, there are very few bacteria in the small intestine, so much so that there is almost no odor at all. However, the large intestine is a different story with approximately two kilograms[10] of bacteria that can easily be noticed by a decent fart after spicy food. The large intestine is a massive fermentation tube.

Gut bacteria helps release ions and other nutrients essential to the body's functions. These are transported into the bloodstream when the colon sucks out the last of the water from the chyme turning it into poop that is dried, compacted, and stored in the *sigmoid colon* and *rectum*.

The body wants to stay as hydrated as possible and it sure as hell isn't going to let valuable water drain out into the toilet bowl, so it sucks it dry as best it can, leaving just enough for the poop to glide out without too much friction.

Here is the fun part: your rectum attaches to your anal canal via a sphincter. Your anal canal is around 4cm[11] long and is met by another sphincter, your bum hole. These two work as a team in synchronization; well, *most* of the time, anyway. Your first sphincter (let's call it the anal sphincter) works involuntarily. Remember, you don't have control of the digestive process still. When it senses the backed-up pressure of the poo in your rectum, it lets out a little sensor sample into your anal canal. Your anal canal then determines whether it's gaseous (a fart) or solid (poo).

Once this happens, your brain gets the signal to let you know which one it is. You are now back in control of your digestive system…or so you think. At this point you know whether you need to find a toilet or just a quiet corner to let off a fart.

Now your bum hole sphincter comes into play. You have a little *sample* that's sitting in your anal canal wanting to come out and, through the sheer miracle of the human body, your brain determines in a split second if it's safe to do so. Your eyes and ears assess your surroundings and your brain pulls up the files (memories) from past experiences to figure out in a micro-second whether or not it's safe to let the turtle out.

If you're in an elevator and you feel that rumble in the jungle, in a split second, your bum hole knows whether it will squeeze shut like your reputation and life depend on it, or if it will risk letting out a squeak, hopefully with no one noticing.

---

[10] Approximately 4.5 pounds
[11] Approximately 1.5 inches

Here's the kicker: if your bacteria has had a hard time trying to digest the terrible food you've given it, or it's having a reaction to something, that little sensor can misfire, giving you the wrong signal and before you know it, you've sharted! So, perhaps think twice about what you eat and don't forget the time it takes for food to get from your mouth to your anus can be up to two days. How hard you party on Saturday night might come back to bite you in the ass on Monday morning at the office or school drop off.

Chapter 4

The Family of Trillions
You Never Knew You Had

*A*s you learned from Digestion 101, there is a large amount of bacteria living in the gut. Before you skip this chapter, you're probably thinking, *So what's the point of this biology lesson and what does it have to do with gluten and celiac disease?*

The answer is everything!

It's vital to understand a little about these itty-bitty tiny creatures that call you home, as the way they live (microbiome) is now being studied as a probable cause of celiac disease, which will be discussed later. These guys need to live in harmony and when they don't, all hell can break loose, which is called dysbiosis. This is a relatively new area of study in celiac disease. So, let me give you a crash course of your extended family. When you learn about gluten, diet, and how it reacts with these little creatures you will have a better understanding of how to heal and keep them happy.

Not many people realize that they have a family of trillions living inside them. Those trillions are *microbes* and without microbes you could not exist. Most people think of microbes or *bacteria* as a yucky thing rather than one of the most amazing elements that make up the human body.

Microbes and the immune system: best friends (most of the time)

Just as you look like a combination of your biological parents' DNA, you also contain the family lineage of microbes from your ancestors[12]. Each of your microbes have their own DNA, so much so that your gut microbes (bacteria) have over 150 times more genes than you. But what does that mean? It means that our microbes contribute more DNA that is responsible for human survival than we do as humans!

Microbes are little itty-bitty unseen creatures that consist of one or just a few cells, and there are more of them living inside you than there are cells in your body. They outnumber the cells in your body by 10 to 1 and make up to 3% of your body weight. For me weighing at 65kg that's 1kg to 2kg of bacteria[13]. And, if they outnumber the cells in your body by 10 to 1, that essentially means that only 10% of you is human cells; the rest of you is microbes. We are more microbe than human. Living, breathing, walking microbes.

One third of your gut microbes are closely the same as everyone else that you know, but two thirds are unique to you much like your fingerprint. They are what make you, *you.*

They live in and on every part of your body, from the inside of your guts and mouth, to your skin, hair, and up your nose. Samples of microbes taken from these various parts of the body show as much diversity of species as you would see in the ocean.

Our gut microbiome contains about 100 trillion microbes made up of more than a thousand different species. One gram of our poo has more microbes (bacteria) living in it than there are humans living on Earth!

The delicate ecosystem

The majority of microbes that call your body home live in the gut. This is important because around 80% of what makes up your immune system is also in

---

[12] Grice E.A. and Segre, J.A. (2012). "The human microbiome: our second genome." *Annu Rev Genomics Hum Genet, 13*:151–170. doi:10.1146/annurev-genom-090711-163814
[13] 143 pounds; 1.43 to 4.29 pounds

the gut. The immune system living in your gut must be able to determine between microbe cells and your human body cells.

Your body is a host to good and bad bacteria. Bad bacteria, despite being called bad, are not always bad. Bad bacteria also have an important role to play. It's very much like the balance in the food chain. Some people think sharks and spiders are bad, yet they play an important role in the circle of life. So do your bad bacteria. Disease begins when the bad bacteria multiply and begin to outnumber the good bacteria.

Nearly everyone routinely carries pathogens (micro-organisms) that can cause disease. Yet, in healthy individuals, the disease does not manifest; rather, the pathogens coexist harmoniously with your good bacteria in a wonderful state of equilibrium. Your good gut bacteria keep control over disease developing, so it's essential to our health and our lives that this stays balanced.

Our microbiome is responsible for our survival just as much as the food we need to live. They have so many diverse jobs, from supplying us with energy, manufacturing vitamins, breaking down toxins, and training our immune system to keep us safe, just to name a few.

Just like the flora and fauna of the Amazon jungle have their own balanced ecosystem, so too does your gut. Overpopulation of one species can upset the delicate balance.

> When there is something wrong with us,
> there is something wrong with our microbiome.

Overpopulation of bad bacteria can be responsible for obesity, depression, chronic disease, and a plethora of other issues. Would it surprise you to know that certain bacteria can be responsible for making you fat?

Now, before you start throwing responsibility out the window for your weight and blaming bacteria, know that what you eat and the lack of exercise is the cause of too much fat-bacteria! How you treat your body can really be the life or death of our precious little critters that make us, us.

Where you're from in the world can also influence which bacteria help you digest different foods. If you're from traditional Asian cultures, you can have more bacteria that breaks down soy in tofu better than someone from a culture that has never eaten it before. If you're from the northern regions of an Eskimo culture, then you host more bacteria to break down whale blubber than most Australians. Just like humans have adapted to live in different environments, our gut bacteria has done the same. And this is passed down through generations.

You may not be able to see your bacteria, but you can feel them and they do a very good job at letting you know when you've pissed them off. The best bacteria in letting you know this is the bacteria that causes diarrhea and vomiting. It's called *salmonella*. Generally, humans have some salmonella bacteria in their stomach and intestines, but our wonderful low pH stomach acid does a good job at killing them off before they have a chance to invade our cells and make us sick.

Most people think of salmonella when they see raw chicken. When properly cooked, the bacteria are killed off. If not cooked properly, then you have probably felt the effects of those nasty critters multiplying inside your body at an exponential rate and biting right into your cells. Without enough stomach acid or the abundance of good bacteria, you're in trouble. Once the cells of the stomach become infected, the cells pump huge amounts of fluid into the gut in an attempt to flush out the bacteria as fast as possible and you then need to empty that. This is diarrhea, that awful, noisy, smelly, and embarrassing bodily function that you just pray for a miracle to stop.

Some people even have what I call a *cast iron gut,* meaning that nearly nothing they eat seems to affect them physically. Just as your microbiome is so uniquely you, so is your response to what you eat. Some people get sick from certain foods and others do not. Take my father, for example. He is going to kill me when he reads this part…but oh well, I think it's funny…

Before I was diagnosed with celiac disease, I was helping my father work on his house one weekend. On a Friday night I purchased fried chicken for dinner. We sat and happily ate what we could. I forgot to put it in the rubbish bin that night and put the leftovers on a trestle outside, completely forgetting about it. Saturday came and went. Then on Sunday I came back from the shops with some food for lunch and my father told me that he'd already eaten.

Puzzled, I asked him what he ate, knowing full well there was no food there. He replied, *"The fried chicken."* I looked at him blankly and said, *"What fried chicken?"* He nodded to the trestle and replied, *"The packet of chicken sitting over there."* *"What the hell, Dad?"* I snapped back quickly. *"You're going to get sick! That's two days old and has been sitting in the sun since Friday!"* He sheepishly shrugged his shoulders and said, *"I thought you must have just bought it. Oh well, it tasted good."*

Needless to say, the old guy didn't get sick. He didn't get bloated. He didn't even fart! Life went on as normal for him. Perhaps he had an abundance of good bacteria on his side.

Microbes are somewhat responsible for your emotions

There are some little critters that can make you feel on top of the world. Your bacteria play a major role in your emotions. Have you ever heard of *serotonin*? It's your natural in-built happy drug. Most people think it comes from the brain, as your brain helps you to express emotion, but 95% of serotonin is produced by the cells of the gut.[14] So, when you're feeling that rush of happiness, you can thank your gut bacteria. It works in reverse, too; when you're feeling depressed, remember that your unhappy gut might be the cause of your unhappy mind.

When you're feeling sick, bloated, tired, and grumpy, this can be your bacteria going spastic, doing backflips, and chucking a tantrum because of what you might have fed it. They are getting pissed off and causing inflammation. On the flipside, you'll know when your bacteria is feeling nice and balanced because you'll touch your flat, calm, unbloated belly thinking to yourself, *Gee I feel good. I feel like I've lost weight.*

Microbes have regular chats with your brain

Your microbiome doesn't just hang out on its own. The microbes throughout your entire body are all interconnected together by the gut and to the brain via a network of nerves, which is now referred to as the *gut-brain-axis*[15]. Your gut-brain (living in your digestive system) seems to be just as complex as the grey matter lump in your head, and the two can talk to each other through a very special nerve pathway that directly links the two together. Kind of like a direct telephone line.

[14] Ormsbee, H.S. 3rd and Fondacaro, J.D. (1985). "Action of serotonin on the gastrointestinal tract". Proc Soc Exp Biol Med., 178(3):333-338. doi:10.3181/00379727-178-42016
[15] Martin C.R., Osadchiy, V., Kalani, A. and Mayer, EA. (2018). "The Brain-Gut-Microbiome Axis." *Cell Mol Gastroenterol Hepatol, 6*(2):133–148.doi:10.1016/j.jcmgh.2018.04.003.

Research suggests that your gut and its chats to the brain are influential on stress, anxiety, and even memory[16].

Have you ever had a *gut feeling* or a strong sense over something? The chemical reactions in your brain are not always responsible for the things you feel or sense but rather a response from the bacteria in your gut that was communicated to your brain.

Your gut needs to talk to your brain. It needs to relay the information of how your body is going. Your brain is quite a distance away from the rest of what's going on in your body and it's not connected to every part, but your gut is. Your gut is the connecting element right in the center of you. It knows what you ate, it knows what's going on in your blood, it's chatting to your other organs constantly, and listening to your cells. All of this information is relayed to the brain for processing. The nerves of your gut reach out to every corner of your body and have such a large surface area that it is the largest sensory organ in your body!

Do you think the brain in your head or your taste buds are solely responsible for why you really *felt* like a steak for dinner? Or you really just *needed* some fresh vegetables? Your bacteria is so connected to what it and your body needs that it has a pretty remarkable way of telling your brain whether or not you need the steak or the vegetables, even without you knowing. But this isn't always a good thing either. If you have too much bad bacteria, these little guys can keep tricking you into thinking you need the bagel and potato chips!

Have you ever had a situation happen that was so stressful that you vomited or had diarrhea? For a long time, I never knew the reason why I would get diarrhea for days and a dry mouth so bad I couldn't eat when I heard the news that a family member had died or there was a serious fight in my relationship. Physical responses like this are a result of your body trying to protect your brain. It eliminates the food in your system via vomiting or diarrhea to conserve energy crucially needed for the brain. Your digestive system requires a lot of energy, so in this instance, your gut determines that your brain needs to survive more than your gut needs food and all resources are diverted.

That's how remarkable your gut is.

---

[16] Forsythe, P. and Kunze, W. (2012). "Voices from within: Gut microbes and the CNS. Cellular and molecular life sciences." CMLS, 70. doi:10.1007/s00018-012-1028-z.

As your microbiome is uniquely special to you, you need to take care of it and know what's best to feed and not feed those lovely little critters. What food you eat on your gluten-free diet can influence how your microbiome reacts and possibly change its structure. People who go gluten-free tend to jump into eating gluten-free alternative food. The problem with this is most of these *alternative* products can cause inflammation and upset the microbiome. Just because you remove gluten doesn't mean your gut bacteria is going to be happy with the replacement. Removing wheat flour from your diet and swapping to pure starches (the bulk ingredient of gluten-free products) is not a healthy diet for your little critters.

Part of healing from a gluten-ravaged body is to balance the microbiome by replenishing your gut with good bacteria and ensure their survival. It's one of the very first things I did when I came off gluten. Knowing that the gut and the microbiome are the center of the universe for my body, it made sense they be the first addressed in trying to help my body to heal. I used a combination of super antioxidants to help remove bad bacteria, enzymes to repair the gut wall, and a super dose of 500 billion bacteria to boost them up. I explain my process in detail in the chapter **My Recipe for Healing the Body**.

Remember: when there is something wrong with you, there is something wrong with your microbiome.

An unhappy gut = an unhappy you.

What the ...!
is Gluten?

Chapter 5

G luten is the collective name for proteins found in all grains like rice, oats, corn, millet, and wheat. In the instance of gluten intolerance and celiac disease, it is the proteins found *only* in wheat, barley, rye, and triticale[17] that appears to activate the immune system, and society refers to these proteins as *gluten*. Gluten proteins in other grains like rice and corn do **not** trigger an auto-immune response for celiac disease. This is especially important to know when you are learning what you can and cannot eat. It's also important if you feel sick from rice to know that it's not triggering an auto-immune response. This could be something else discussed a little later.

In Latin, gluten means *glue* and that's what it does; it's the glue that binds wheat products together. Gluten is responsible for the elasticity of wheat products, like a pizza dough for example, and it reacts amazingly well with oxygen for dough to expand.

Spotting a gluten-containing grain can be tricky sometimes. Wheat, rye, and barley have a wide variety of other names and forms, so below are 21 other names to be wary of:

[17] A hybrid of wheat and rye

Tricky Names for Wheat		
Atta	Graham	Tabbouleh
Bulgur	Kamut	Triticale
Cous Cous	Matzah	Triticum
Durum Wheat	Matzoh	Wheat Bran
Einkorn	Seitan	Wheat Germ
Farina	Semolina	White Flour
Frumento	Spelt	Whole Wheat Flour

Let's put the wheat protein (gliadin) under the microscope

Think of protein like a long chain of pearls joined together. When it's eaten, the body snips up the protein into small chunks of pearls called *polypeptides*. The body has special enzymes that then pick off each pearl one by one for processing. These individual pearls are called *amino acids,* which get absorbed into the blood stream. These amino acids are the building blocks for the cells in our body.

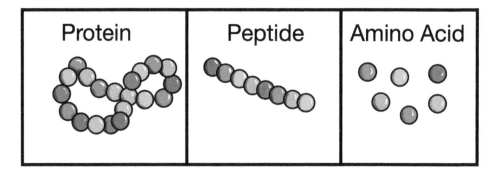

However, wheat protein (including rye and barley) is a whole different story. We don't have the special enzyme to break down the wheat protein-pearl-chain into individual pearls (amino acids) to be used by the body. The body instead tries to digest these long peptide chains, and mostly they don't get processed properly and are pooped out. Some, however, do make their way into the bloodstream and can cause all sorts of havoc. The main culprit is the peptide pearl clump called *alpha gliadin*. Alpha gliadin is the main protein to which celiacs react. This little bad boy is made up of a select group of amino acids and has a special code written across it. Let's name this code *Gliadin Fraction 9*.[18] In the later chapter Celiac Disease Uncovered, I'll show you how your body locates this little code in the food you eat and sets off a chain reaction.

Wheat in its original whole form, oddly enough, was once upon a time somewhat nutritious. It's made up of the Bran, the outer layer protective shell which contains vitamins and minerals and is high in fiber. Inside the Bran is the Germ, and it contains all the nutrients that can give life to a new plant. It also has more vitamins, minerals, fats, and so on. Then there is the Endosperm. This is the carbohydrate rich part of the grain and contains protein. It's a balanced grain overall, but as you'll read later on, commercial baking typically does not use the whole grain anymore.

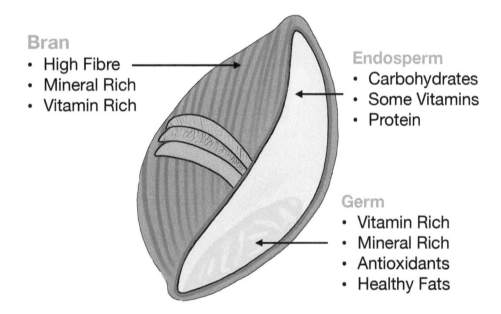

Bran
- High Fibre
- Mineral Rich
- Vitamin Rich

Endosperm
- Carbohydrates
- Some Vitamins
- Protein

Germ
- Vitamin Rich
- Mineral Rich
- Antioxidants
- Healthy Fats

The wheat grain was designed by nature to have a defense mechanism, also known as an anti-nutrient. They are compounds built within many plants and are designed to protect the plant against fungi, pests, and even animals while growing.

---

[18] Cornell, H.J. and Maxwell, R.J.. (1982). "Amino acid composition of gliadin fractions which may be toxic to individuals with coeliac disease". Clin Chim Acta, 123(3):311-319. doi:10.1016/0009-8981(82)90176-0

They prevent the plant's healthy nutrients from being absorbed properly when it's eaten and can have a toxic effect. Then, over time, this teaches the animal who's eating it, "This stuff is making me sick so I won't eat it anymore," thus the plant species can survive. It reminds me of the yucky nail paint my mother put on my fingers when I was a child to teach me to stop biting my nails. When I would stick my fingers in my mouth, it would release a foul bitter taste and over time I stopped biting my nails.

This defense mechanism in plants is called *lectin*.[19] In wheat, the lectin is called *wheat germ agglutinin* (WGA).[20]

That's good for the plant, but the problem is lectin can be toxic, not only to pests and animals but humans too! Lectins have been found to cause inflammation, which is a key factor discussed in a later chapter, **The Bonnie & Clyde of Your Guts**. It can get past the gut wall and inside the body where it can deposit in various organs. Many lectins can be cooked or soaked out and the body can be good at blocking these lectins with our own version of a defense mechanism—various types of sugars and enzymes—but this doesn't always work to plan.

Dr. Perlmutter, Dr. Grundy, and Dr. Tom O'Bryan talk about how lectins (like WGA from wheat) can cause inflammation, interfere with gene expression, cross the blood-brain barrier, bind to activate white blood cells, induce cell death, disrupt endocrine function, and can cause gastrointestinal upsets. You can read more about this on their sites, blogs, and published books.

Not only does wheat have gluten, it has the lectin WGA. When the body is not optimal, *our* defense mechanism doesn't work very well against the plant's defense mechanism. There's on-going study of the effect that lectins have on the body and more research is showing the link between lectins and auto-immune diseases.[21]

When people switch to a gluten-free diet, typically the consumption of rice and corn increases as these can make up the main ingredients in gluten-free food. The

---

[19] Freed, D.L. (1999). "Do dietary lectins cause disease?". *BMJ, 318*(7190):1023–1024. doi:10.1136/bmj.318.7190.1023

[20] Pusztai, A., Ewen, S.W., Grant, G, et al. (1993). "Antinutritive effects of wheat-germ agglutinin and other N-acetylglucosamine-specific lectins". Br. J. Nutr., 70(1):313-321. doi:10.1079/bjn19930124

[21] Vojdani, A. (2015). "Lectins, agglutinins, and their roles in autoimmune reactivities". Altern. Ther. Health Med., 21 Suppl 1:46-51. Retrieved from: https://www.ncbi.nlm.nih.gov/pubmed/25599185

increased consumption of these alternate grains also increases the consumption of lectins, and people still report ill health on a gluten-free diet.

While lectins from grains can cause inflammation in various parts of the body (including the brain) and some symptoms can *appear* the same as a gluten-reaction, only gluten from wheat, barley, and rye has the ability to cause the auto-immune response of celiac disease.

To understand gluten better, let's look at the history of wheat

It only makes sense, considering celiac disease and NCGS (Non-Celiac Gluten Sensitivity) are digestive disorders, that we would want to understand not only the cause of this disease, but also why we have it. Maybe the answer is written in history.

Tens of thousands of years ago, we hunted and gathered our food, hence the term *hunter-gatherer*. We required some serious energy expenditure to hunt and catch wild game, and we foraged for hours through vegetation growing wild all over the land.

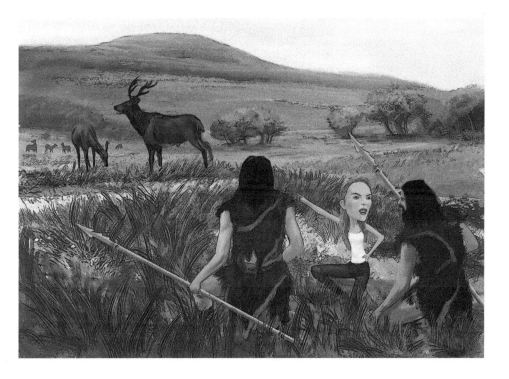

The game and vegetation were organic—untouched and nutrient dense. In the hunter-gatherer days, gluten intolerance was not an issue because wheat did not exist.

Approximately 8,000 to 10,000 years ago, humans began the agricultural era of domestication and growing of grains, grasses, and vegetables.

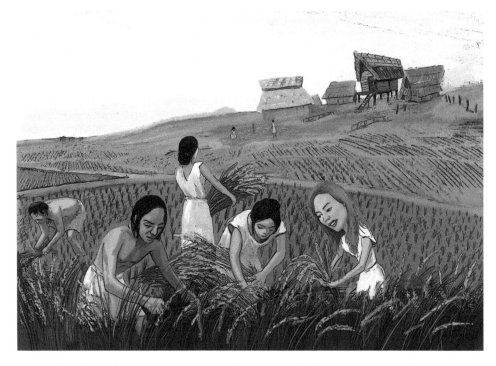

So far, there doesn't seem too much wrong with this picture yet, right? Sounds like a good idea that we could stay in one place longer and not have to roam so much to find food.

But keep in mind, we are not designed to break down wheat proteins into perfect amino acids to be absorbed by the body, and lectins can be toxic.

So, how did our ancestors eat wheat and not get sick?

To start off with, the whole grain was used and ground down to a flour consistency, which included the bran (outer layer) and the germ (seed) and endosperm (starchy carbohydrate) components. The enzymes in the bran and the germ played a role in helping to break down the gluten protein that is contained within the starchy endosperm.

The flour was then fermented. Our ancestors would take several days to make a loaf of bread because yeast didn't exist. Instead, they used a sour culture that would not only help the dough rise but also help break down the gluten and the lectins in the dough to make the bread more edible and *somewhat* more digestible.

I once heard a story of an Italian family that had a starter sour culture that was over 100 years old. Every time they made bread, they would remove a portion of the culture to add to the dough and then add back to the culture to keep it fermenting and growing. In fact, you can continue to maintain and use the same starter culture forever, and this Italian family passed it down through generations. Imagine what magical power of the ancient bacteria culture could impose upon the wheat protein, not to mention how flavorful the bread would be.

The original wheat varieties didn't yield many grains per stalk, therefore there wasn't as much flour produced. However, moving forward another few thousand years you'll find that farmers began to select the best yield of their crops to re-plant the following season to create a stronger more nutritious food supply. Ok, still not such a bad idea, however, with this selective breeding comes the larger portion of gluten protein being present, along with the larger portion of everything, including the lectin.

So, now we have a larger portion of protein in the grain, more toxic lectin, stronger crops yielding more, and more people are eating it than before.

"How did our ancestors eat wheat and not get sick?" Who says they never got sick?

Aretaeus of Cappadocia[22] was regarded as the second greatest medical scholar after Hippocrates and lived sometime around the 2nd century BCE. He wrote many volumes of information surrounding medical conditions (known today as a thesis) that went unknown till his work was rediscovered around the middle of the 16th century CE. In 1552, one thesis titled "On the Causes, Symptoms and Cure of Acute and Chronic Diseases" was published in Latin. He described many clinical conditions of diseases and recorded accounts of epilepsy, pneumonia, tetanus, asthma, uterine cancer, and various kinds of insanity. He also recorded the earliest accounts on diphtheria, heart murmurs, and…celiac disease!

---

[22] Tekiner, H. (2015). "Aretaeus of Cappadocia and his treatises on diseases". *Turk Neurosurg*, *25*(3):508-512. doi:10.5137/1019-5149.JTN.12347-14.0

So, it would seem that a few thousand years ago, things began to change and reports of celiac disease continued through the ages and into the 1800s.

Where the process of food changed

Louis Pasteur,[23] a French chemist and biologist known for the discovery that germs cause disease, also discovered a new secret process in the mid-1800s that would change the way bread would be made forever. *Pasteurization!* Which in turn yielded yeast! Yeast has now replaced the fermented starter culture that was once used with a more readily available baker's yeast. Today, it's called instant dried yeast.

The early 1900s saw the start of the Industrialized Food Revolution. Many of the famines and food problems during WWI, WWII, and the Great Depression began to ease with the incorporation of advanced agricultural machinery, factory assembly lines, refrigeration, and transportation.

During WWII, governments began to invest heavily into the mass manufacture of packaged foods that were easily transported and shelf stable to feed the soldiers, as so many were malnourished. This was known as a K-Ration, and was a small boxed set of three portions of shelf stable food to provide breakfast, lunch, and dinner. The person responsible for this product was Dr. Ancel Keyes.

This sparked a revolution.

Food was now being produced on a mass scale. However, it was in the mid-1900s when cross genetic breeding and splicing began. Food became a *product* that was grown *faster,* yielding *more,* and costing *less.* Perhaps—maybe in the very initial stages of this change toward modifying food—the intention was for good, to feed a growing and starved population during war times. However, nowadays, it appears to be all about big profits for big companies and the health of the people seems of no consequence anymore.

They sold us on the idea that this method of modifying food was to produce higher quality, better tasting, longer lasting, and more nutritious food. However, what we were left with *was* better looking *but* less nutritious, tasteless *food-like*

---

[23] Barnett, J. (2000). "A history of research on yeasts 2: Louis Pasteur and his contemporaries, 1850–1880". *Yeast, 16*(8):755-771.

substances. These modifications begin in the labs by hybridizing and genetically modifying the strains before planting, then after each crop, repeating the process again and again trying to perfect the strain. Perfect it for size and color, and protect it against pests, disease, and degradation; all things that occur naturally in farming. This new process applies itself to most mass-manufactured produce and grains today.

The original wheat stalk species known as Einkorn is a mere shadow of its former self and is rarely used in commercial baking at all now. Most people have never heard of it or tasted it, and probably never will, me included.

Unfortunately, the whole grain and stone milling method is hardly used anymore and deemed impractical for commercial use. A roller mill invention took its place and uses cylindrical rollers to break off the bran and the germ. What's left is the starchy endosperm portion of the grain. But why? Why remove all of that natural nutrition and helpful elements to breakdown gluten?

The simple answer is, it's not an effective shelf stable product. The germ contains oils, which make stone ground grains spoil over time as the oils go rancid.

What happens to the bran and the germ when it's removed? Well, it's fed to animals in feeding lots, and sometimes put back into the bread marketed as an *added nutrient!*[24]

They feed the bran and germ to animals? That can't be good, can it?

Cows are designed to eat sprouted grass. Their four-chambered stomach allows them to break down grass but not grains. In feed lots where cows consume a grain-based diet, there are tons of reports of acidosis, infections, and abscesses which could be caused by gluten, and the grain in general.

Rather than taking days to prepare through fermentation, commercially made bread can be prepared and packaged in as little as two hours. All the anti-nutrients and irritants are still in there. Some wheat is even specifically grown to have an even larger portion of gluten in it marketed especially to commercial bakers.

Essentially, wheat has become a toxic, inflammatory product.

---

[24] "Cereal germ". Retrieved from: https://en.wikipedia.org/wiki/Cereal_germ ; "Enriched flour". Retrieved from: https://en.wikipedia.org/wiki/Enriched_flour

Fast forward to today

Agriculture became monoculture. Today in most animal farming, cows are only farmed with cows and not other animals. In grain farming, corn is only grown with corn and not other plant species. What this does is remove the circular balance of life. Bacteria mixes and fertilizations from fauna and the reliance of species working together to create food is now gone. For example, cow manure contains vital bacteria, and is a fertilization food source for plants and the earth. If there are no cows rotated around on harvested crops, where do the soil and plants get nutrients from? If you plant some species like Marigolds (flowers) next to vegetables, they ward off pests, but many of these practices are gone now, which means artificial use of pest management is required.

Long gone are the days of having to fight or forage for your food.

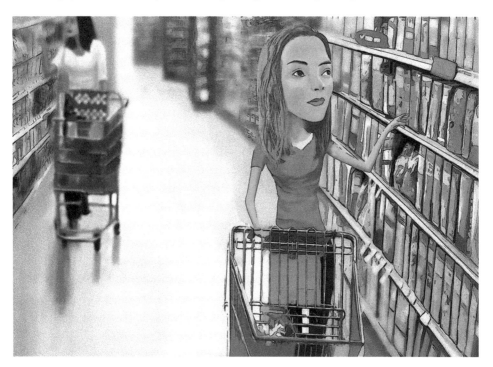

Now we can just step inside an air-conditioned grocery store and load up a cart full of whatever our taste buds desire.

No more needing to grow our own food in our backyards and eat what's in season; we can eat a mango all year round if we please. But where does it come from, what's being used to make it grow, and how long has it been stored is a whole other story.

The USA is one of the largest producers of wheat in the world.[25] However, much of it is bred to withstand the massive doses of pesticides, herbicides, and fungicides sprayed on them time and time again. Some grains have now become patented products!

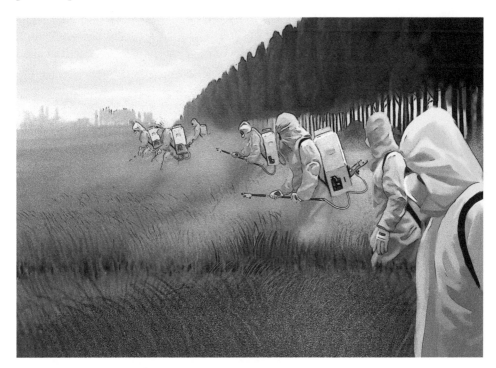

Have you ever heard of Round-Up™? That amazing poisonous weed killer that you may have used in your garden? Well, that product is made by a company called Monsanto (who also manufactured the warfare chemical Agent Orange). Did you know that the main ingredient in this product is glyphosate, which is an herbicide chemical that is applied to broadleaf plants and grasses to kill it off? I've used Round up in my garden before to kill weeds. One drop on a weed and the plant is dead days later. Glyphosate is toxic to humans and it says so on the packaging. However, Monsanto has engineered crops to withstand being sprayed with Round-Up, known as *Roundup Ready Crops*.[26] They can spray this chemical

---

[25] World Agricultural Production. (2020). *Wheat Production by Country 2020/2021.* Retrieved from: http://www.worldagriculturalproduction.com/crops/wheat.aspx

[26] "Roundup Ready". Retrieved from: https://en.wikipedia.org/wiki/Roundup_Ready

directly onto the plant and surrounding soils to kill off the weeds around it, *but not the plant itself.*

Do you really think it's safe and natural for us to be eating grains from a Round-Up ready crop? Stephanie Seneff, a research scientist at MIT and Anthony Samsel another research scientist of Agricultural Chemicals, have concluded a study with suggestive evidence that Glyphosate may play a role in the development of celiac disease. They discuss how glyphosate can imbalance the gut bacteria, inhibit special enzymes that are important for detoxification, and cause depletion of amino acids (special protein compounds), which all are associated with celiac disease.

Today's wheat crops can have multiple applications of chemicals from start to finish. These range from:

- chemicals in the germinating phase to make them sprout
- chemicals in the growing phase to make the stalks stronger
- chemicals to make them yield more
- chemical treatment in the factory when processed

Our soils are so depleted and sterile of micronutrients, trace elements, and minerals to make plants grow that we now need to use chemicals to do the growing instead, all the while killing our planet. How can you grow a healthy plant in sick soil? What we have now is a cascading effect of land degradation, high-yielding-chemical-maze food crops, nutrient deficient food, destruction of the atmosphere from toxic gases, and the destruction of other land areas where they have to dispose of by-product chemicals.

Dr. Peter Greenlaw talks about how our soils are so bankrupt of nutrients that you would need to eat 12 apples in 2009 to get the same nutrient value of 1 apple in 1976.[27] Spinach would require 51 bowls to get the same benefit of 1 from 1957. If this really is true, then it's baffling to think how much our soil has been depleted of nutrients over time from constant injection of chemicals, and the continuous harvesting and re-harvesting without letting the soil regenerate.

---

[27] Greenlaw, P. and Harper, D. (2015). "America's 'Polluted' Diet". Retrieved from: https://www.linkedin.com/pulse/americas-polluted-diet-peter-greenlaw-dr-dennis-harper-peter-greenlaw

Not only did this food change come about for vegetation but also animal farming.[28] For example, chickens are grown to maturity in 1/3 the natural time and are yielding 400% more meat in 2005 compared to 1957. They are being fed these modified grain products and are put on *fattening* diets before slaughter for rapid weight gain to yield more dollars per pound.

If you're a celiac and react to ingesting gluten, could eating a steak from a cow that's only been fed gluten-containing grains be affecting you? So far, there seems to be no conclusive evidence that cows who are fed grain in their diet can cause an auto-immune response in celiac disease patients when we eat the meat. But what we do know is that inflammation is caused by this unhealthy grain fed meat and excess consumption of it can still cause much harm to the body in other ways.[29]

Do you drink cow's milk? Did you know that, in the 1950s, the average yield of milk per cow was around 5,300 lbs compared to today's average yield of over 20,000lbs?[30] How do you think those cows can produce nearly three times as much milk as they were originally designed, not to mention what chemicals and hormones are passed down to the milk?

My point to all this is: think back to the hunter-gatherer days, what they would have eaten, and how they got their food. Now think about the changes over the last few hundred years, especially the last 50 years. Know and understand that the consumption of what was once wild natural food became selected food, became modified food, and now isn't really food anymore.

What do you think happens to the body when it's not designed to digest wheat proteins and processed de-natured chemical concoction food-like products? Things start to go wrong! The body malfunctions and some of these problems can be passed on to our generations through our genes. Celiac disease is passed through our genes from our ancestors as discussed in the chapter **Celiac Disease Uncovered**. On average, although the life expectancy of our ancestors was shorter,

---

[28] Zuidhof, M.J., Schneider, B.L., Carney, V.L., Korver, D.R., and Robinson, F.E.. (2014). "Growth, efficiency, and yield of commercial broilers from 1957, 1978, and 2005". Poult Sci., 93(12):2970–2982. doi:10.3382/ps.2014-04291

[29] Ponnampalam, E., Mann, N., and Sinclair, A. (2006). "Effect of feeding systems on omega-3 fatty acids, conjugated linoleic acid and trans fatty acids in Australian beef cuts: potential impact on human health". Asia Pacific Journal of Clinical Nutrition, 15(1):21-29. Retrieved from: https://www.drperlmutter.com/study/effect-feeding-systems-omega-3-fatty-acids-conjugated-linoleic-acid-trans-fatty-acids-australian-beef-cuts-potential-impact-human-health/

[30] O'Hagen, M. (2019). "From Two Bulls, Nine Million Dairy Cows". Retrieved from: https://www.scientificamerican.com/article/from-two-bulls-nine-million-dairy-cows/

I believe their bodies were stronger, denser, and healthier than the average person today.

What do you think the health of our children's children will be like in the future? Our future generations may have a shorter life expectancy than us. Not longer. So the scales have shifted in reverse possibly for the first time in history. The CDC in the USA has released research showing a decline in age expectancy already just between 2016 to 2017.[31]

Today, most people sit on their bums for an hour commuting to work, sit at their desks all day for eight hours, commute back, then sit at home in front of the TV at night for another few hours, eating food that came from a packet, that was processed in a factory, and grown in a lab. Whoosh, take a breath! (I was no exception to this either.)

Just to push the point even further and scare you into eating healthy, the top leading causes of death in the United States and Australia are heart disease and cancer, which can result from on-going chronic *inflammation* (a modern-day disease you will learn about in later chapters). In 2016, the CDC recorded that 1 in 4 Americans will die from heart disease, but I think that number has grown closer to 1 in 3 people as the CDC predicts this to be the case by 2050.

We are a far cry from the days when our ancestors were up at dawn fetching firewood, loading the wagons, hunting for food, and washing our clothes by hand. *We are using less energy but consuming more.*

Humans went from being healthy, strong individuals thousands of years ago, to starving and diseased during war times and only two generations later, we have an obesity epidemic on our hands.

It is my belief and opinion that selected breeding, hybridization, modification, chemicalization, and a down-right stuffing up of the food system (combined with lack of physical movement) is why we are getting fatter, sicker, and more diseased.

---

[31] Arias, E. and Xu, J. (2019). "United States Life Tables, 2017". National Vital Statistics Report, 68(7):1-66. Retrieved from: https://www.cdc.gov/nchs/data/nvsr/nvsr68/nvsr68_07-508.pdf

Chapter 6

Starvation
To Dietary Requirement

How and why did wheat go from a solution to starvation to its role as a government-issued dietary requirement?

The story begins with Kellogg's Corn Flakes.

Dr. John Harvey Kellogg (1852-1943) was a medical doctor, surgeon, and nutritionist. He ran a sanatorium[32] in the USA and treated his patients with a holistic approach using exercise, hydrotherapy, sun-bathing, colonics, and abstention from smoking, alcohol, and even sex.

He practiced the religious views he preached, adopted seven children, and never engaged in sex with his wife. Dr. Kellogg also believed that masturbation was an illness of the mind to be cured with a healthy diet. He was a vegetarian and a promoter of a grain-based diet over meat. Together with his brother, Will, they developed a few flaky grain-based cereals, one of which was corn flakes, and they fed these cereals to the patients at the sanatorium to treat their sexual illness.

Kellogg's early work in raising awareness of food's impact on health was quite profound. Whether or not the use of cereals was beneficial to treating mental illness, his work was instrumental in understanding food's impact on gut flora and the development of diseases from an imbalanced gut microbiome. He believed that a poor diet increased harmful bacteria in the gut that could affect other parts of the body, and that changing the gut flora would alleviate disease.

---

[32] A medical establishment for the treatment of chronic illnesses

However, original intentions seem to change when profits are involved. His brother wanted to keep the corn flakes recipe and process a secret, but John didn't share those views and let anyone into the sanatorium to see how they made this revolutionary product. One observer was C. W. Post, who copied the process of grain-based cereals and went off to start his own company, which made millions of dollars.

I believe the Kellogg boys were a driving force behind changing the breakfast diet forever, from meat and eggs to grain-based cereals with skim milk.

The brothers began to argue over the addition of sugar to the corn flakes recipe. John was against it and Will was for it, which sparked a decades-long feud. Will went off to start his own cereal company in 1906, which then became the Kellogg Company around 1930.

Throughout the Great Depression, people were starving, so this product was instrumental in providing readily available calories in the form of a shelf stable product. Project forward to today and we have a clear example of good intentions gone bad, as now nearly all of our calories are from shelf stable products!

Will's company was one of the first to put nutrition labels on food and offer an inside-the-box prize for children. His marketing efforts really started to take off. As the company grew, so did the refinement of its products. They became less nutritious and more shelf stable.

The era of false and misleading information

Over the next few decades, there was a drop in cardiac death, and here Dr. Ancel Keys (the same guy that invented shelf stable K-rations for the Army soldiers) enters the story. His theory? The reduced consumption of saturated fat from meat and eggs was responsible for the drop in cardiac death. His *belief* changed the world as we knew it.

Ancel Keys was a lover of education, so much so he studied chemistry, economics, political science, zoology, oceanography, biology, and physiology. But did all this study really make him the expert of human nutrition?

Ancel was the originator of the hypothesis that saturated fat causes heart disease. He was convincing in his theory that saturated fat was responsible for all the ill health in the world and he needed a way to back up his beliefs. He researched the link between fat and cardiac death from 21 countries but chose to only publicize the results from the seven countries that confirmed his theory, leaving out the other 14! Essentially, he completely fabricated his evidence, yet it got worldwide recognition.[33][34]

The wheels were in motion for more consumption of packaged carbohydrate foods, and companies were coming out with even more interesting ways to hook the consumer.

Over the next few decades, cardiac death continued to rise, but why was this true if people were eating less saturated fat? Refined carbohydrates and sugars increased and recent studies have found this to be the culprit, *not* saturated fat.[35]

It was in 1977 when consuming wheat became a dietary guideline pushed to every household in Europe, USA, and Australia. This all began because of the McGovern Report[36] which published that the American people should reduce their risk of a heart attack by reducing their intake of cholesterol from saturated fats. Ancel Keys' fabricated data provided the foundation to change the world, and not in a good way.

Scientists challenged these reports, saying that there was no scientific evidence to suggest this correlation. Dr. Robert Olsen of St. Louis University pleaded for more research on this subject before making public announcements. Senator McGovern stated that they didn't have the luxury of time to perform such research! The McGovern report apparently was written by the senator's young staff member, with no background in nutrition or medicine, who happened to be a vegetarian.

Apparently a few select staff from the USDA,[37] also with no background in health sciences, believed in this McGovern Report and wanted to make it a nationwide policy that fat was bad. By sifting through scientists and finding one who would agree with them, they eventually achieved their goal. To keep the ball

[33] Banerjee, A. (2018). "The Diet-Heart Hypothesis: Changing Perspectives". Perspectives in Medical Research, 6(2):4-11. Retrieved from: http://pimr.org.in/benerajee-vol-6-issue-2-2018.PDF
[34] Aseem, M. (2013). "Saturated fat is not the major issue". BMJ, 347:f6340. https://doi.org/10.1136/bmj.f6340
[35] DiNicolantonio, J.J., Lucan, S.C., and O'Keefe, J.H. (2016). "The Evidence for Saturated Fat and for Sugar Related to Coronary Heart Disease." *Prog Cardiovasc Dis.*, 58(5):464–472. doi:10.1016/j.pcad.2015.11.006
[36] United States Senate, Select Committee on Nutrition and Human Needs, *Dietary Goals for the United States*, 1977, Washington: US Government. Retrieved from: http://hdl.handle.net/2027//uiug.30112023368936
[37] United States Department of Agriculture

rolling, they had to *convince* other scientists to agree with their report and what better way to do it than with the probability of halting government funding for the scientists.

In the early 1980s, Luise Light, a nutritionist teaching at a university in New York, was hired by the Department of Agriculture to create a new food guide to replace the four basic food groups system that was already being used.

Luise and her team designed a pyramid that was based on vegetables, fruits, and limited starches. They submitted it to the USDA for approval, but when Luise saw the finished product she realized it was ***not*** what she'd submitted. Luise then found out the changes made by the USDA were to garner the support of big agriculture companies in the food industry.[38] Perhaps the lining of pockets continued.

Luise's original guideline recommended 5 to 9 servings of fresh fruits and vegetables a day was replaced by 2 to 3 servings a day. Her original recommendation of 3 to 4 servings of carbohydrates per day was swapped to a whopping 6 to 11 servings a day, and the list went on.

Despite Luise's objections to this altered version of the pyramid, the government still released it. Luise made it very clear that this guideline would lead to an obesity epidemic and here we are today with 1/3 of all Americans and Australians experiencing obesity and prone to heart disease, cancer, and diabetes.

Australia released a food pyramid in 1982, a decade before the USA, modelled off a 1974 Swedish version. Again, the consumption of wheat was to be a primary source of calories. I'm sure we've all seen a picture of the food pyramid. Do you remember what was at the bottom to be eaten in the largest quantities? Wheat!

---

[38] Light, L. (2004). "A Fatally Flawed Food Guide". Retrieved from: www.whale.to/a/light.html

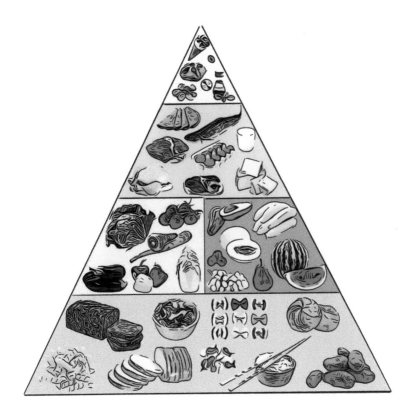

The dietary guidelines have been revised today, using different methods to display the correct balance of the food categories. But guess what? Refined carbohydrates still remains one of the largest portions.

Could you imagine what would happen across the western world to all those agricultural companies if everyone suddenly made refined carbohydrates only 10% of their diet? Profits would plummet and no big Ag company will stand for that. So, in my opinion, I assume the lining of government officials' pockets continues and the people get a revised excuse for a food guideline that is only marginally better than the original from the 80s.

Big Ag companies and politicians are not the only ones to blame for increased consumption of wheat. Would it surprise you to learn that your brain is one of the biggest culprits in this matter?

Chapter 7

I Was Getting
High Off My Bread

*I*s bread comfort food or the next best drug to opium?

It's 6 a.m. before work in winter, and I've just sliced myself a hot, fresh piece of bread and slathered it with honey. *Gee this tastes good.*

It's Sunday and I'm sick with the flu, so I eat a piece of toast with Vegemite to settle my stomach and give me some nourishment. *Ahh, I feel better now.*

It's Wednesday night, stew night. But I need some bread to soak up the juices. *This just feels so comforting.*

It's date night and I've just picked up a loaf of artisan bread to have with my quince paste and blue cheese. *This flavor is really setting the mood.*

It's friends-over-for-a-meal night and we've served up a loaf of Italian garlic bread and bruschetta. *How nice it is to share bread with friends.*

It's I'm-in-a-rush-for-lunch day and I'll grab a salad baguette. *Perfect, this will tide me over.*

I'm sure you can get the idea here, every time I ate bread:

I felt good!

I felt great!

I felt nourished!

I felt satisfied!

I felt whole!

I felt healthy!

No wonder I kept eating it.

I thought that was all normal. Normal to love bread, normal to experiment with recipes, just normal. But as it turns out, I might have been getting a little *high* each time I was eating bread.

I love coffee and I drink coffee because I know it wakes my brain up in the morning and makes me feel more energized. *(Terrible, I know)* But I understand the effects of caffeine on my brain and I continue to consume it with purpose. I do the same thing with wine. I drink wine knowing that I will get a relaxed buzzed feeling and I'll probably get a little chatty, too.

So why couldn't I put two and two together with bread?

Being an asymptomatic celiac, I lived a life not knowing that bread was destroying my body. I never *felt* bloated from bread so I didn't realize the effect it had on me till I quit cold turkey.

While my body crumbled as I detoxed from the gluten, turns out my brain was also detoxing from the drug-like addiction it had to gluten.[39] Your brain has morphine receptors in it, the same that bind to opiate drugs to elicit the effects of getting high.

Even though we can't digest gluten protein properly, sections of the gluten-protein-pearl necklace (peptides) still get into our bloodstream. Once these sections of protein are in the bloodstream, they can pass through the blood-brain barrier which is a special cheese cloth lining designed to keep toxic substances out. Once these peptides get through that protective barrier, they can bind to morphine receptors. Wheat is exceptionally unique in this ability to bypass the blood-brain barrier as that does not happen with other grains like millet or flax.

This polypeptide reaction in the brain is called *exorphin*. I was getting high off my bread! I was getting a form of mild euphoria every time I ate bread and it worked so well that it had me coming back for another hit day after day. This exorphin effect can be so profound that it has the ability to mask its own toxicity and the harmful gastrointestinal upsets for some who are asymptomatic.

---

[39] Pruimboom L. and de Punder, K. (2015). "The opioid effects of gluten exorphins: asymptomatic celiac disease." *J Health Popul Nutr, 33*:24. doi:10.1186/s41043-015-0032-y

This exorphin effect of wheat on the brain can be blocked if you take opiate-blocking drugs *or* stop eating wheat. So, if opiate-blocking drugs work, then this backs up the very real effect gluten has on the brain. People who are administered opiate-blocking drugs report feelings of withdrawal, and the same can apply when you stop eating wheat. This is exactly what happened to me; I was *coming down* and having withdrawal symptoms for months from this drug-like effect that had been going on in my brain for the best part of 30 years.

The relationship between gluten and the brain is so alarmingly unique that multiple studies indicate a large number of schizophrenia patients show great improvement in behavior, and less side effects from drugs when gluten is removed from the diet.[40] Children suffering from ADD/ADHD also show many signs of improvement when gluten is removed from their diet.[41]

Do I recommend that people with celiac disease wean themselves off wheat to avoid the withdrawal symptoms? I'm not a doctor and can't give any advice; you will need to make up your own mind but let me throw in some food for thought.

Everyone is different. People may not have such severe withdrawal symptoms like I did, and some may even have worse. Wheat can have an undeniable hold on the brain. It can be so powerful that if one tries to slowly cut back on gluten, they may continue to make up excuses to have another sandwich or one last bagel over and over again. How many times have we said, *"I'll go to the gym tomorrow, or I'll start that diet tomorrow"* and tomorrow takes forever to come?

If someone is diagnosed celiac, then the smallest trace amount of gluten can prevent the gut from healing, continue to cause malabsorption and gastrointestinal upsets, and the list goes on.

In my opinion, I believe that going through whatever withdrawal symptoms may happen is a better approach than trying to wean off gluten as I believe the ongoing brain and intestinal damage is far worse, even from the smallest amount of gluten. I'm glad I ripped the band aid off. I just wish I had known what was going on so I was better prepared mentally for the challenge. It would have been

---

[40] Levinta, A., Mukovozov, I., and Tsoutsoulas, C. (2018). "Use of a Gluten-Free Diet in Schizophrenia: A Systematic Review. Adv Nutr., 9(6):824–832. doi:10.1093/advances/nmy056
[41] Niederhofer, H. (2011). "Association of attention-deficit/hyperactivity disorder and celiac disease: a brief report." *Prim Care Companion CNS Disord, 13*(3):PCC.10br01104. doi:10.4088/PCC.10br01104

nice to know there is a real chemical reaction happening and I wasn't just losing my mind.

It's interesting to watch someone eat bread now with this new knowledge. I watch with bated fascination at my husband's orgasmic reaction when he bites down into his ancient grain sourdough bread. I'm not sure if I feel sorry for his brain-faked reaction, or slightly jealous.

Chapter 8

Gluten

Is Lurking in What?

What was supposed to be a naturally occurring protein found in a few food sources has now been extracted, processed, combined, mutilated, and added into many other products on the market shelves today…and not just food.

Would you be surprised if I told you that some vitamins contain gluten? Or your household cleaning products? I bet you'd fall off your chair if I said to you that bath and body products like your shampoo, face cream, and makeup can contain gluten.

Also, you should probably be a little wary next time you go to mail the annual Christmas cards and lick the back of the envelope to seal it, or even lick the stamp. Yes, they can contain gluten. On your journey to discovering where gluten is hidden, don't be surprised if you find that your first three to four visits to the shopping center take twice as long.

My husband gave up on accompanying me to the shops in my early celiac days, as it usually ended up in him getting frustrated because I was taking so long to choose products. Then I would get upset that he wasn't being *'supportive enough.'* Then we'd have an argument that I was acting like a little bitch. Turns out this was mainly because of my mood swings from the gluten withdrawal I didn't know I had.

So, the word from the wise is, go it alone!

Back then, I started at one end of the shopping center and snaked my way around, I was reading the back of labels on almost everything, including products

I rarely buy. Much to my surprise, it seemed that gluten or gluten derivatives were in over half of the products on the shelves.

Common products where gluten is lurking

Most people who think of wheat can relate it to breads, pastas, bagels, etc. Below is a list of the most common foods made of gluten in some form or another, just to give you a recap.

Common Foods Comprising of Gluten		
Bagels	Cous Cous	Muffins
Bread	Crackers	Pasta
Cakes	Croutons	Pastries
Cereal	Crumbed Food	Tortillas
Cookies	Deli Salads	Wraps

Breakfast cereals

Most breakfast cereals are made with wheat and if they are made with corn or rice, they may have gluten added or are processed in a facility where wheat cereals are made, thus cross contamination is likely. You will find many of the major cereal brands below to show you that many contain gluten as a main ingredient. They are pretty obvious to see when you read the ingredients, and then there are others, for example, like Rice Bubbles that contain a barley malt extract (which is gluten too) but is not so obvious as it doesn't contain the ingredient wheat. A point to note with products is that they can change ingredients over time, and maybe one day there might be a gluten-free version available.

Common Breakfast Cereals containing Gluten		
All Bran	Frosted Flakes	Raisin Bran
Bran Flakes	Fruits Loops	Rice Bubbles
Cheerio's	Granola	Special K
Coco Pops	Just Right	Sultana Bran
Corn Flakes	Milo Cereal	Sustain
Corn Pops	Muesli	Weet-bix
Crunchy Nut	Nutrigrain	Wheat Chex

Uncommon products where gluten is lurking

Beverages

A word on alcohol. You can buy gluten-free alcohol, beer especially, but navigating the world of spirits is a different story. Although vodka, whiskey, and bourbon are usually made from gluten-containing ingredients, experts believe that the gluten is removed during the distilling process thus rendering it safe for Celiacs. However, everyone can react differently, and the bottom line is that those products are still made with gluten. There is so much controversy surrounding spirits and whether or not they cause a reaction, and some people can be more sensitive than others. Without even thinking, one night I had a gin and mineral water, later on that night I was on the couch sick and feeling terrible. It was only one glass. I could not work out for the life of me what it was, so I spent the next day recounting everything I ate, not thinking of what I drank. Randomly, I decided to check the bottle of gin. I'd never really had gin before so I never thought to look. Sure enough, it's made from gluten-containing grains! Another thing to remember is that there are so many fun new drinks coming out on the market, and although the main ingredients might be gluten-free, be wary if they have any flavors or additives in the mixes. When looking and testing for spirits, perhaps a trial may be needed or just choose an alternative. I personally love vodka with some kombucha and have found an amazing vodka made in Japan that's distilled from rice, so it is a great example of an alternative.

Cheese

Some cheese has bread mold added to the cultures to ferment it. This mainly accounts for blue cheese, but with some research, I'm sure you can find a good brand that uses other cultures so you don't miss out.

Snack bars

These were my go-to for work. I'd run into the store and grab a box of muesli bars and use these as my mid-afternoon pick-me-up. When more companies jumped on the bar-bandwagon, awesome and healthier alternatives were coming out that I wanted to try. Problem is, even some of the best brands still use wheat derived products and when they don't, there can be the issue of cross contamination. Many snack bars can contain oats, and plain old oats are a no go- at this stage, as I explain in the later chapter **To Oat Or Not To Oat.** So, it's best to look for a gluten-free brand until you understand more about ingredients and how to navigate what really contains gluten vs. what product is covering it's butt from cross-contamination. I recommend Zego who offer contaminant-free, allergy friendly snack bars.

Snack food, sauces & condiments

Here is the really tricky part about hidden gluten. The extraction and chemical change it has undergone has now made it an entirely new ingredient with new names.

It lurks in items as colorings, fillers, and flavoring agents, maltodextrin (usually corn-derived but also can be from wheat), hydrolyzed vegetable protein, extenders, emulsifiers, textured vegetable protein, and so on. You don't want to be secretly glutening yourself, so I would strongly suggest staying away from products that have these types of ingredients anyway. They are highly processed chemical concoctions that bring you no health benefits anyway, so why eat it?

Here is an example of sneaky gluten: I picked up a packet of liquid bone broth to make a soup with. Naturally, I would think bone broth would be nothing but bones and vegetables, yet in the fine print, there was gluten hiding under 'Caramelized Sugar (from Wheat). This was not a product to which I would have guessed companies would add gluten containing additives. At the time of writing, I am 4 years diagnosed and would like to think I'm pretty good at spotting products on a shelf with gluten. Yet even at this point, I find surprises, and this goes to show you can never assume. Companies are coming out with new products all the time so there probably will be no end to reading labels and double checking everything for the rest of our lives unfortunately.

Uncommon Products Where Gluten is Lurking		
Atkins Snack Bars	Deli Meats	Ovaltine
Battered Fish	Dressings	Pies
BBQ Sauce	Dumplings	Play Doh
Beer	Envelopes	Potato Gems
Bloody Mary Mixes	Fish Fingers	Potato Wedges
Blue Cheese	Flavoured Coffee Syrup	Quaker Bars
Bone Broth	GNC Snack Bars	Rice Crackers
Burger Patties	Gorgonzola Cheese	Roasted Nuts
Canned Soup	Grain Chips	Roquefort Cheese
Carman's Snack Bars	Gravy Powder	Seasonings
Celebrity Slim Bars	Hoisin Sauce	Soy Sauce
Cheap Vitamins	Ice Cream	Spring rolls / Pot stickers
Cheese Spreads	Kellogg's Snack Bars	Stamps
Chewing Gum	Liquorice	Stocks / Stock Cubes
Chips	Lollies	Supplements
Chocolate	Malt Liquor	Sushi
Cliff Snack Bars	Mayonnaise	Teriyaki Sauce
Corn Chips	Medications	Uncle Toby's Snack Bars
Crisps	Milo	Vegemite Spread
Crumbed Snacks	Nature Valley Bars	Vegetarian Meats

The key to the products in the table above, is that while they are highly susceptible to containing gluten, there are brands that don't contain gluten. So yes, you can still eat ice cream, chocolate, and chips, but it just takes a little practice and time to find out which ones. Unfortunately, you are no longer able to buy what product you want based on how awesome the front of the packaging looks. We now have to wear our geek hat and read labels constantly.

Health products

Cheap vitamins, medications, and mineral supplements can use gluten in the coatings and casings. Gluten can also be used as a filler and labeled with tricky names. A study in 2011 investigated the presence of gluten in 21 common supplements and the results showed gluten present in 23.8% of those samples.[42] This makes it just a bit more challenging for those following a gluten-free diet. If you are unaware of the exact ingredients on medications and vitamins, there is a chance you could be getting glutened and hindering your ability to maintain a healthy gluten-free lifestyle.

Women love Vitamin-E. Vitamin E tablets and Vitamin-E in our skin creams. Would you be surprised if I told you that a significant source of Vitamin E is wheat germ oil. Remember that lovely Wheat Germ we learned about before that contains natural oils that can spoil flour? It's a rich source of Vitamin E. Typically, it's thought that the refinement process of wheat germ oil removes the gluten, but are you willing to take the risk when there are better alternatives out there?

I had a bout of random headaches during some stressful weeks at work and took some Aspro Clear™. I rarely took painkillers but checked the ingredients and thought nothing of it. A week later I was chatting to some ladies on my Facebook group about gluten in medications, and one of them said she was accidentally glutening herself by using a different brand of Aspro. I was shocked and darted to my packet to check again; sure enough, mine was fine, but hers was not.

So, please always make sure you: 1) spend a little more money on a reputable brand for these products, 2) check the labels, and 3) speak with the pharmacist to ensure that any medications given do not contain gluten or its derivatives.

---

[42] Oancea, S., Wagner, A., Cîrstea, E. and Sima, M. (2011). "Gluten screening of several dietary supplements by immunochromatographic assay". Roum Arch Microbiol Immunol, 70(4):174-177.

Bath & body products

At the start on my gluten-free journey, I didn't even realize that some of my bath and body products contained gluten. I have been lucky enough for the past 10 years to be very organically minded and have always tried to use only natural products, primarily because of my skin's super sensitive nature from my childhood dermatitis. But I didn't know that gluten was hiding in them too.

There is much debate around body products that contain gluten and whether it affects celiac disease patients. So far, I haven't been able to identify any research that shows that there is a link between using gluten-containing products and the degradation of the intestinal walls from a stimulated immune system. However, there are countless claims from celiac patients who report adverse side effects to these products in some form or another. The most common is an acute irritation to the skin may be possible for some and can be linked to the aggravation of dermatitis. However, is that attributable to gluten ingredients or could it be to other toxic chemicals too?

Some people have reported that repeated exposure over a long period seems to present a build-up in the body and lead to the overall feeling of ill health. There is some literature that shows a link between inhaling the vapors of gluten containing product and the negative effects on the body. Either way, products that contain gluten-derived ingredients are not needed when there are better alternatives available.

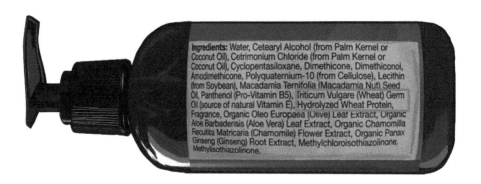

Ingredients: Water, Cetearyl Alcohol (from Palm Kernel or Coconut Oil), Cetrimonium Chloride (from Palm Kernel or Coconut Oil), Cyclopentasiloxane, Dimethicone, Dimethiconol, Amodimethicone, Polyquaternium-10 (from Cellulose), Lecithin (from Soybean), Macadamia Ternifolia (Macadamia Nut) Seed Oil, Panthenol (Pro-Vitamin B5), Triticum Vulgare (Wheat) Germ Oil (source of natural Vitamin E), Hydrolyzed Wheat Protein, Fragrance, Organic Oleo Europaea (Olive) Leaf Extract, Organic Aloe Barbadensis (Aloe Vera) Leaf Extract, Organic Chamomilla Recutita Matricaria (Chamomile) Flower Extract, Organic Panax Ginseng (Ginseng) Root Extract, Methylchloroisothiazolinone, Methylisothiazolinone.

I was standing in the shower one day, soaking up the hot water on a cold winter's night. I took my time reading the labels on the back of my shower products, just out of pure curiosity. Sure enough, there it was. One of them had wheat germ oil and hydrolyzed wheat protein. What on earth could be the benefit from putting this in my shampoo? Apparently, it's very nourishing for the hair. It stunned me to say the least. Then I went on the hunt throughout the bathroom. I'm glad to say, for the most part, my bathroom was free of these hidden gluten nasties. Thank you, organic products.

However, for people who buy their products from the supermarket rather than a health shop, you will probably find that gluten is present in quite a few of them, along with myriad other ingredients you won't be able to pronounce and probably shouldn't be using. I've been a big believer in using very natural products and the idea of putting silicones, plastics, and chemicals that make vehicle fuel on my body makes me shudder. These are all excess toxins that your body is not designed to absorb. Most women don't even realize their face cream contains parabens which can disrupt their hormone and endocrine system. Gluten in lipstick and lip balm is another one to be wary of. Remember this rule: *what goes on the lips gets eaten.*

So, enough of my ranting. Here is a list of where gluten is hidden. Go get yourself a rubbish bag and get cleaning.

Bath & Body Products that may contain Gluten		
Baby Powder	Hair Masks	Shampoo
Bath Salts	Hair Oil	Shower Gels
Body Lotion	Lip Gloss	Sunscreen
Conditioner	Makeup	Sun Tan Creams
Face Cream	Mouthwash	Toothpaste

Overall, what's the rule? When in doubt, leave it out!

Chapter 9

Celiac Disease
Uncovered

You may have heard some people refer to themselves as celiac, gluten-sensitive, gluten intolerant, non-celiac gluten-sensitive, and so on. But what is the difference between these terminologies?

Gluten related disorders break down into three categories.

- non-celiac gluten sensitivity
- wheat allergy
- celiac disease

To understand how these disorders affect the body, we need to understand a little about the immune system. Your immune system is your inbuilt defense mechanism against pathogens (bacteria and organisms that can cause disease), viruses, toxic chemicals, and basically anything that can cause the body harm. Your body has four special groups of immune systems. One each in the brain, the liver, the blood, and the largest one in your gut.

These groups have sets of warfare soldiers. They are broken down into five categories and each of them have their own unique training and deploy to a particular pathogen or foreign invader. The technical name for the warfare soldiers is *antibodies*, and they each have a special code name and a type of pathogen they are trained to eliminate.

Non-celiac gluten sensitivity (NCGS)

Non-celiac gluten sensitivity is the more clinical name for what people call gluten-sensitive, or gluten intolerant.

When you consume gluten-containing foods the body sees clumps of those protein pearls in the digestive system and has a hard time trying to break them down properly. The acute reaction that people feel from this is called non-celiac gluten sensitivity.

People can have varying degrees of reactions but sometimes the body responds like this:

Uh-oh human host, you shouldn't have fed me that food. Now I will make you bow down to the toilet bowl and vomit like a hung-over teenager, or make it come out of your rear end just as profusely. Perhaps I'll plug up your bum hole so you can't poop for a week or make you feel bloated and downright miserable for a while.

Once your body has finished punishing you for feeding it gluten, the lesson is over until the next time you consume gluten.

However, some people may not have an acute reaction but rather present with a problem that's totally unrelated to the gut, like sore joints, brain fog, migraines, rashes, or eye problems but have no clue it may be linked to gluten consumption. These responses are called *inflammation* and they usually target the weakest spot in the body.

The other thing to consider is that testing for non-celiac gluten sensitivity doesn't rely on a medical scale; the only way to diagnose is to eliminate the wheat and see if your problems go away.

Non-celiac gluten sensitivity is appearing to affect quite a wide range of the population, with Dr. Alessio Fasano (a guru in the celiac disease world) believing that upwards of 6% of the US population could be struggling with gluten.

But wheat also carries that lectin called WGA, so how do you know if you're reacting to the lectin or the gluten? Gluten and WGA are two very different things that can affect the body. I guess it doesn't matter either way. If you feel better when you don't eat wheat, *then don't eat it.*

Wheat allergy

This is where some of your warfare soldiers come into play.

In the instance of a wheat allergy, your IgE Warfare Soldiers are sent into battle against what it thinks is the foreign invader. These soldiers then bust out sub-soldiers called *histamines* and they cause an inflammatory response to deal with the allergen. The type of allergen will determine the reaction you have. Typical responses may be swelling of the throat, lips or tongue, wheezing, coughing, red eyes, and vomiting. However, to add to this, you may also present any of the symptoms in the non-celiac gluten sensitivity category.

Your IgE soldiers also get activated in other circumstances as well, not just wheat. To give you an example, a pollen allergy might cause a runny nose. A fur allergy might cause you to have swollen, bloodshot eyes, and a rash. Those reactions are caused by your histamines trying to purge the toxic substance out of your body. There is no one size fits all rule. In some cases, some people can have an anaphylactic wheat allergy that will require them to carry around an Epi pen, just as one might for nuts. You can have a wheat allergy without having celiac disease, or you can have celiac disease without a wheat allergy, or if you're really unlucky you can have both.

A simple blood test can test for elevated levels of IgE and will let you know if you are allergic to wheat or any other potential allergens like pollen and dairy.

Celiac disease

This is *not* an allergy or a sensitivity. It is a disease, a *real* disease, just like any other. It falls within the category of auto-immune disease.

When you eat wheat, your immune system has detected those clumps of protein pearls (peptides), and in most cases, has recognized the common *gliadin* pearl clump. Your immune system recognizes a special code (in most instances it's gliadin fraction 9) stamped on the peptide clump, just like a virus protection software detects an incoming threat from the internet. The body then busts out your different set of Warfare Soldiers; these bad boys are called IgA and IgG. These guys have special training to defend against real threats like viruses, but for some reason, they have detected that code on the gliadin clump of pearls, become confused, and decided it's a foreign invader that needs to be eliminated. This is *not* a good thing. This is *not* supposed to happen, and in a normal functioning body, this does not occur.

When you eat wheat, those warfare soldiers get their wires crossed and, thinking that wheat is a bad thing, rush down to your intestines to deal with the bagel and cream cheese you ate for breakfast. They are going nuts down there, lighting fires to burn out the gluten.

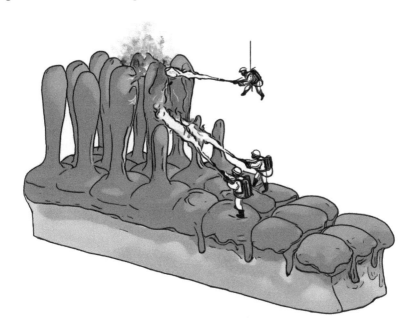

Instead of giving those poor guys a rest and time to retreat, you eat a ham and salad baguette at lunch. So, now they are back and calling for reinforcements with the blow torches and really going crazy in effort to eliminate gluten.

Then you get home from work and, with any luck, your loved one has surprised you with a special dinner. They looked up a recipe on Pinterest (because you keep raving about this app) and they've made a sumptuous lasagna for dinner.

Repeat this process for most meals of the day, for most days of the week, for most weeks of the month, for most months of the year, and for most years of your life.

At this point, your immune system is in overdrive. It's saying, *"F* you"* and is blasting everything...including the lining of your intestines. It's burning the whole place down to the ground. As you learned from Digestion 101, this is where all those beautiful villi live that absorb nutrients into the body. Those soldiers have turned from antibodies into *autoantibodies*. They are not only attacking the gliadin pearl group (gliadin fraction 9) they are attacking your own body tissue on autopilot.

This defines an auto-immune disease. Your immune system is wrongly activating on autopilot. Somewhere along the line in your life, your body shifted balance and triggered your antibodies to recognize gluten as a bad thing, one this trigger occurs, those soldiers are reprogrammed for life and there is no going back. I discuss a bit further on the possible different triggers.

Now, when you eat gluten, the fire never goes out. Those poor soldiers are exhausted. How well do you think they can do their job when you get a real virus attack on your body or infection? Have you noticed that you get the cold or flu more frequently now and it lasts for longer periods? Your immune system is so overworked that it's not able to protect the body like it should.

Now your body is struggling to regenerate. Your intestines are torched to a smoldering, raggedy sausage casing. Your immune system is sick, there is no villi left, and you're struggling to absorb nutrients from food.

Just how much gluten does it take to destroy the villi?

It only takes a very small amount of gluten to set off your immune system and cause damage. In fact, the amount is so small it's recorded through studies that 50 milligrams of gluten[43] is enough to do the job. How much is 50 milligrams you might ask? It's roughly 1/70th of a slice of bread. That's all that it takes to start the erosion of your precious little villi. If you continue to have that kind of exposure after approximately 90 days, your villi will be all gone.

Everyone reacts differently to gluten and so far, the '*acceptable*' level of gluten intake seems to be at 10 milligrams where intestinal damage does *not* occur. To put that in perspective, 10 milligrams is 1/350th of a slice of bread. However, everyone reacts differently and everyone will have a different tolerance level, but there is not a lot of difference between 1/70th a slice of bread 1/350th.

---

[43] Cohen, I.S., Day, A.S., and Shaoul, R. (2019)."Gluten in Celiac Disease-More or Less? *Rambam Maimonides Med J.*, *10*(1):e0007. doi:10.5041/RMMJ.10360

If you're celiac, you should probably come to terms with the fact you pretty much can never consider eating gluten again. I couldn't imagine trying to cut up a piece of bread into 350 squares just to get a hit!

Once your villi are gone, your intestinal wall starts to have holes in it where larger un-processed food particles and toxins can get into your bloodstream. This is called *leaky gut* and is explained in the chapter called **The Bonnie & Clyde of Your Guts**.

You may have an acute response from eating gluten but that is just the tip of the iceberg. Underneath that is the ongoing chronic battle that's affecting your organs, not just your intestines. This condition is called inflammation and affects so many other parts of the body from your joints to your brain.

Inflammation = Disease

One of the unfortunate factors with an auto-immune disease is that once diagnosed, if not managed correctly you may be at a higher risk of developing other auto-immune diseases. A Danish study[44] in 2016 revealed auto-immune diseases were more prevalent in celiac disease patients (16.4%) as compared to the general population (5.3%). It just so happens that type 1 diabetes is one of the most common auto-immune diseases associated with celiac disease patients.

It remains unclear whether celiac disease directly leads to other auto-immune diseases, but my belief is chronic inflammation does. When the body is in a constant state of inflammation it's called *systemic inflammation* which is the chronic activation of the immune system.

Will a gluten-free diet be the answer? Well, that depends. Many of the gluten-free alternative foods available are unhealthy and can also cause inflammation, feeding the fire so to speak. Even though you may not activate your warfare soldiers by not eating gluten anymore, you can still cause inflammation from the other unhealthy foods you eat.

---

[44] Grode, Bech, Jensen, et al. (2018). "Prevalence, incidence, and autoimmune comorbidities of celiac disease: a nation-wide, population-based study in Denmark from 1977 to 2016." *European Journal of Gastroenterology & Hepatology, 30*(1): 83-91.

Conditions linked with Celiac Disease		
Addison disease	Epilepsy	Multiple Sclerosis (MS)
Amenorrhoea	Gastro Intestinal cancers	Osteoporosis
Arthritis	Hashimoto's thyroiditis	Sarcoidosis
Autoimmune hepatitis	IgA nephropathy	Sjogren's syndrome
Chronic Liver disease	Lupus	Type 1 Diabetes Mellitus

There are around 100 auto-immune diseases recorded so far. Below is a list of the most common auto-immune diseases that have been associated with celiac disease.

Level 1 - Acute Symptoms (Immediate response to Gluten)		
Bloating	Itchy Skin	PMS
Brain Fog	Joint Pain	Sleepiness
Constipation	Migraines / Headaches	Stomach Cramps
Diarrhoea	Mood Swings	Tingling in Hands/Feet
Fatigue	Mouth Sores	Vomiting
Gas	Pale Foul-smelling stool	Weakness

Symptoms of celiac disease

Below I've broken down the most common symptoms of celiac disease into two categories: acute and chronic. People can have slight degrees of symptoms or so many of them I can't believe how they have managed to get through life. There are even symptoms that are not on this list.

Inflammation from gluten can manifest itself in almost any area of the body and cause any type of symptom.

Level 2 - Chronic Long Term Symptoms (Ongoing response to Gluten exposure)		
Anxiety	Endometriosis	Lactose Intolerance
Chronic Fatigue	Failure to Thrive	Low Immunity
Delayed Puberty	Fatty Liver	Malabsorption / Anaemia
Dental Cavities	Fibromyalgia	Neuropathy
Depression	Infertility	Recurrent Miscarriage
Dermatitis / Eczema	Irritable Bowel Syndrome	Un-explained weight gain/loss

One of the most common symptoms of celiac disease is nutrient deficiencies. This makes total sense. When there are no villi left, how well can we absorb nutrients? The main deficiencies are iron, vitamin D, vitamin B12, folate, magnesium, niacin, and zinc. People may have one or a few of these nutrient deficiencies. For me it was only iron.

I am what they call asymptomatic (someone who does not present any acute symptoms) so I didn't have an acute response to eating gluten, which is why it was the last thing on my mind in terms of what was wrong with me. I had, in-fact, several level 2 severe symptoms: dermatitis, dental cavities, endometriosis, infertility, low immunity, and malabsorption/anemia. But I had no idea they were linked to celiac disease. I was dealing with all these issues separately, not knowing there was a singular underlying cause. Was it a blessing that I didn't get acutely sick from gluten, or a curse?

Now for the big finale.

If left untreated, celiac disease can lead to cancer,[45] and lymphoma cancer happens to be the most common for celiac disease patients.

[45] Silano, M., Volta, U., Mecchia, A.M., et al. (2007). "Delayed diagnosis of coeliac disease increases cancer risk". *BMC Gastroenterol, 7*:8. doi:10.1186/1471-230X-7-8

Why do you and I have celiac disease but others do not?

The most widely used answer is genetics. However, like everything, there is always a grey area.

Turns out there are genes for celiac disease and it's recorded that around 40-50% of the population carry these genes. Carrying the gene does not guarantee that you will develop celiac disease, it just means that you have an increased susceptibility to it. Roughly 1 in 40 gene carriers will develop celiac disease.

In celiac disease patients, either one or both of the associated genes[46]—HLA DQ2 and HLA DQ8—are present. The HLA DQ2 gene imparts a greater risk of celiac disease over DQ8.

I have the HLA DQ2 gene.

As of 2020 in the United States, 1 in 133 has celiac disease and of those, 97% of them are undiagnosed. In Australia, 1 in 100 has celiac disease and about 75% are still undiagnosed.

Is genetic predisposition a case of the chicken and the egg? If it's genetics, how did it become a genetic problem in the first place? It must have started somewhere and there is a growing number of people being diagnosed with celiac disease now more than ever. Here's my explanation.

Are you born with celiac disease? No, you are not. You're born with the gene. I have celiac disease now, so how did I get it if I wasn't born with it? This is such a good question, and essentially it comes down to an over-responsive immune system coupled with a change in *environment.* Remember that shift of balance I described earlier that flipped a switch?

---

[46] Tye-Din, J., Galipeau, H. and Agardg, D. (2018). "Celiac Disease: A Review of Current Concepts in Pathogenesis, Prevention, and Novel Therapies". Front. Pediatr. Retrieved from: https://www.frontiersin.org/articles/10.3389/fped.2018.00350/full

Studies implicate a range of environmental factors can be a trigger, and the change in gut microbiome[47] [48] is one of them. Something shifts the balance from gluten-tolerance to a gluten-reaction.

The change in environment can happen at any stage of your life, whether you're a two-year-old child or 60-year-old adult. The environment change *could* be triggered by early and excessive use of antibiotics, trauma, infection, stress, a major emotional event, health degradation, other diseases, or other auto-immune diseases.

The other perception is simply wear and tear. Your warfare soldiers simply malfunction after years of repeated gluten exposure.

You generate a whole new body's worth of cells every seven years. Some take longer to turn over and others regenerate very quickly. The mouth, as you learned from Digestion 101, turns over cells super quick; that's why it can heal so fast. The same is true for your intestines. Those cells that line your villi and your gut can shed old cells and grow new ones somewhere between three to seven days.

That's great, but it's not if you eat toast for breakfast, a baguette for lunch, and pasta for dinner every day. Repeat that gluten-filled cycle over and over again, year after year, and your poor little intestinal cells are getting damaged constantly, they just can't regenerate fast enough to keep you safe. That special lining of the gut gets torn so many times your body says, "*Stuff you, I give up.*"

When celiac disease is activated, it's like winning the auto-immune disease lottery. There is no rhyme or reason as to why I have it but my mother does not, or you have it but your friend does not. Something has simply activated it, and that's it.

When I look back at my life, I believe something happened when I was a young child around the age of four, which is when dermatitis showed up. It stuck with me into my teens, followed by endometriosis problems in my 20s, then anemia into my 30s. Working my way back down the line of symptoms, it became clear that I'd been suffering for a long time. But what initially caused the trigger? I don't

[47] Chander, A.M.,, Yadav, H., Jain, S., Bhadada, S.K., and Dhawan, D.K.. (2018) "Cross-Talk Between Gluten, Intestinal Microbiota and Intestinal Mucosa in Celiac Disease: Recent Advances and Basis of Autoimmunity." *Front Microbiol,9*:2597. doi:10.3389/fmicb.2018.02597
[48] Cenit, M.C., Olivares, M., Codoñer-Franch, P., and Sanz, Y. (2015). "Intestinal Microbiota and Celiac Disease: Cause, Consequence or Co-Evolution?" *Nutrients, 7*(8):6900–6923. doi:10.3390/nu7085314

know; I don't really remember being four! Maybe a round of strong antibiotics early on triggered it. Maybe it didn't. Maybe when I electrocuted myself by sticking a screwdriver in a wall socket caused the imbalance. Maybe it didn't. Maybe it was the muddy creek water I drank on the farm? Who knows…The annoying part about this trigger is that once it's happened, there is no going back and switching it off. You now have celiac disease for life!

Oddly enough, 1 in 500 people with celiac disease have selective IgA deficiency.[49] This means that these people make very low levels of these types of warfare soldiers. We need them to fight infection in the mucus membranes of the body, which are pretty much everywhere.

People with IgA deficiencies may get recurring infections. IgA deficiency can be linked to arthritis, lupus, and celiac disease (all auto-immune diseases.) There are more recent studies now showing that early testing of children for IgA deficiency can help lead to early detection of Celiac and other related diseases.[50]

Turns out I am IgA deficient too. I hit the auto-immune jackpot!

How to diagnose for celiac disease

The fool proof way to determine if you have celiac disease involves the following:

1) blood tests (celiac serology)

2) endoscope with a biopsy of the intestines

3) genetic test

Blood tests are the ideal starting point to see if your antibodies are being triggered. This test is called *transglutaminase IgA antibody* (tTG IgA).

For a more accurate diagnosis, the deamidated gliadin IgG (DGP IgG) antibodies should also be included. I know that sounds like a mouthful to say, but

---

[49] Kumar, V., Jarzabek-Chorzelska, M., Sulej, J., Karnewska, K., Farrell, T., and Jablonska, S. (2002) "Celiac disease and immunoglobulin a deficiency: how effective are the serological methods of diagnosis?" *Clin Diagn Lab Immunol,* 9(6):1295–1300. doi:10.1128/cdli.9.6.1295-1300.2002
[50] Bienvenu, F., Anghel, S.I., Besson Duvanel, C. et al. "Early diagnosis of celiac disease in IgA deficient children: contribution of a point-of-care test". BMC Gastroenterol, 14(186). https://doi.org/10.1186/1471-230X-14-186

if you're concerned about celiac disease, consult your doctor about a celiac lab test that covers tTG IgA and DGP IgG.

There are two problems with celiac serology tests: they can throw false-positive results and false-negative results.

If your villi are only half-way worn down, there is a chance that the test results will come back saying that you are negative for celiac disease. Uh oh. Could you end up walking out of the doctors with celiac disease and be told you're fine and to keep eating wheat? Possibly. This is a false-negative result. Being IgA deficient (like me) can also throw a false negative result, so coupling the test with deamidated gliadin can help achieve a more accurate result.

If you already have other types of auto-immune diseases—type 1 diabetes, liver disease, Hashimoto's disease, and even arthritis—you can test positive when in fact you ***don't*** have celiac disease. That's why it's important to get the two tests performed together.

Some testing labs don't have the capability to test for all sections of the gluten protein. Remember that gluten is like a pearl necklace and it gets broken up into long clumps of pearls. Most labs can only test a few common chunks of these pearls (codes stamped on them) and the most common of them is the gliadin fraction 9 clump. People can react to different chunks of pearls and if the right ones don't get tested, sometimes test results can come back with a negative reading.

The other thing that can give a negative test result is if you're not eating gluten. When I was first diagnosed, my tTG IgA levels were at 'greater than 80' then 18 months later after eliminating gluten, they were 'less than 3.' My IgG levels went from 'greater than 242' to 'less than 5.' So, the summary on my follow-up blood test after 18 months of not eating gluten said, *The presence of celiac disease is very unlikely, less than 5% chance.* Does this mean I've cured my celiac disease? No, it will always be there; it's just gone back to being dormant because I'm not activating my immune response by eating gluten.

So, if someone was already on a gluten-free diet but not yet diagnosed celiac, they would have to start eating gluten again to get tested. Would you want to do this? Most people who are comfortable on a gluten-free diet would never dream of eating gluten again just to get a diagnosis. What purpose would that serve? To confirm that they shouldn't eat gluten, which they aren't doing anyway? You would be surprised to hear how many people are faced with this question from a doctor. The only thing it would do, would be to confirm how strict you would have to be if you were positive.

Are you living a gluten-free lifestyle and haven't been diagnosed with celiac disease, but every few months with friends you will eat a pizza, and think *"it's ok, it's only once and a while?"* or you are not fully educated and hidden gluten really is in your diet? If you are considering you may have celiac disease and are not strictly adhering to a gluten-free diet like your life depends on it, then are you doing yourself an injustice?

An endoscope is the only fool proof way to see if your intestinal lining is being damaged. When an endoscope is performed, a small biopsy of the intestinal wall is taken and analyzed under the microscope to see if your villi are damaged, be it great or small.

The five levels of your villi and how they are measured

When biopsies are evaluated, there are markers that define the stages of degradation of your villi. They are mostly divided up into five stages, but how this is reflected on reports varies between countries. Some countries list the results as a 'marsh' score, and other countries like Australia, simply write the description of the result.

Stage 0

In a healthy person the villi would be a stage 0. Meaning the villi appears to be normal and there is no evidence of lymphocytes (immune defense white blood cells) infiltrating the villi.

Stage 1

Epithelial cells are a special lining of the intestinal wall. They are joined together by tight junctions that make it a relatively impermeable membrane. They are essentially the special cells that line the villi. In Stage 1, lymphocytes are present and can indicate inflammation and the potential for damage. When you have *'increased intraepithelial lymphocytes,'* this is an indicator of developing celiac disease but it doesn't always mean celiac disease. Increased lymphocytes can indicate food intolerances, Sjogren's Syndrome, and Irritable Bowel Syndrome (IBS).

Stage 2

Think of the villi like the fingers on your hand. At the base in between your fingers is a section called a *crypt*. More lymphocytes are present in Stage 2, along with bigger depressions than normal in the crypts between the villi. When the crypts are larger than normal, it's called *crypt hyperplasia*.

Stage 3

Stage 3 is a combination of 1 and 2 (increased lymphocytes and large crypts) as well as the flattening of the villi. This is known as *villous atrophy*.

There is *partial atrophy*, meaning the villi are still there but smaller; there is *subtotal villous atrophy*, meaning the villi have shrunk significantly; then there is *total villous atrophy*, meaning there is no villi left at all.

Stage 4

This stage is mostly present in older people with celiac disease. This is where the villi are not only totally atrophied, but the crypts in between have shrunken as well.

What a recovering biopsy looks like

I had my second biopsy exactly 18 months after my first one. It wasn't necessary, but I wanted to see what was going on inside and to see if my villi were healing as expected. I'd been working my ass off with food, exercise, sun, and supplements from the day I was diagnosed. I needed to know my plan was working so I asked for a second biopsy and this was the result:

Specimen Report: The sections show fragments of small intestinal mucosa with preserved villous architecture. There is intraepithelial lymphocytosis. No parasites or granulomas are identified. There is no evidence of epithelial dysplasia or malignancy. Summary: intraepithelial lymphocytosis consistent with treated celiac disease.

The first thing I saw when I read this report was *'preserved villous architecture.'* Yippee, there they are. **My villi are back!** So, this meant that I was at a Stage 1 instead of 3 and 4.

Genetic testing is important because if you test positive to the genes, but negative to serology and/or biopsy, you are still at risk for the disease as you go on in life. Remember that 1 in 40 people who carry the gene develop celiac disease and there is no rule as to if or when it gets activated.

If you get these tests done knowing that you feel sick from gluten, and your results come back that your intestines are fine, you're in luck. You're what's called *non-celiac gluten-sensitive* or if your IgE antibodies have flagged in your blood test, then this means you have a gluten/wheat allergy. Both of these results are the best you can hope for. This means that you do not have the auto-immune disease that is destroying your intestines. You simply react with an inflammatory response to gluten and that's it. If you test negative for the celiac gene, then you will most-likely never develop the disease.

If you find you get quite ill in some form when you eat gluten, celiac or not, then much of this book still applies to you in terms of how to live a life without gluten.

If you get shitty news like me, that your intestinal villi has suffered atrophy, then welcome to the Celiac Journey.

The iceberg gets deeper

The average person can wait years to be correctly diagnosed with celiac disease. The Celiac Disease Center at the University of Chicago Medicine reports that the average length of time it takes for a person to be diagnosed with celiac disease in the US is 4 years. For others, it can be much longer. Why so long? There are several reasons for this:

- People are getting false-negative blood results and do not pursue a biopsy.
- Some of us don't present the usual intestinal upsets so some doctors think there's no additional screening needed.
- Many doctors may not be aware of the prevalence of celiac disease and the various other symptoms outside gastrointestinal upsets or associated diseases.

Educating doctors is one way we can speed up the process. I've heard countless people say they had to practically yell at their doctor to order a celiac test and sure enough, they had celiac disease. I would have been diagnosed much earlier if my general doctor had screened me for celiac disease when I was anemic, as this is one of the major markers. But they didn't know.

Even as individuals we can help speed up the process to achieve a diagnosis for others. Imagine you now know about the acute and chronic symptoms of celiac disease and your friend mentions to you that their child is suffering from brain-fog, dermatitis, and feeling sick from food. I'm not saying that celiac disease will always be the cause, but it's a good starting point to rule out. Maybe even my own life would have been different if someone had told me that anemia is a symptom of celiac disease.

Many doctors wouldn't even think to associate gluten with being the cause of joint pain, an odd skin rash, eyesight problems, fatigue, or brain fog. Many gynecologists are also not aware of the role that celiac disease plays in infertility. People seek treatment for these symptoms individually not knowing there may be a connected underlying cause. If gluten isn't the underlying cause, then inflammation may be.

It seems sometimes that doctors just dole out drugs left, right, and center for treatment of the presented ailment, not the cause. And here begins the snowball effect.

You take the drugs to *ease* the symptom.

The drugs can upset the gut microbiome.

Other symptoms/side effects develop.

Now you're back at the doctor's trying to get more drugs for other newly developed issues. All the while, the *cause is not being treated* and you continue to stay on the merry-go-round.

If I have celiac disease will other family members have it too?

A first-degree relative (parent, sibling, child) of a celiac disease patient has about a 75% chance of having the gene, but remember, only 1 in 40 gene carriers will develop celiac disease.

Getting your family members tested may not always be so easy. The last thing anyone wants to hear is *"I have a disease. You should get you tested to see if you have it too."* Once you know and understand the signs and symptoms of celiac disease, obviously you want to see if anyone in your family is concerned with those issues before bringing it up, and if so, talk about your experience and knowledge and the simplicity of a blood test to start. Various celiac organizations around the world have official letters that can be taken into your local doctor. It describes the prevalence of celiac disease, why the patient is requesting the tests, and what tests are needed.

My mother has many auto-immune diseases and complained about stomach upsets. I pleaded with her to get tested and her response was that she simply didn't want to know. I continued to hound her and eventually she gave in and got tested while still consuming a gluten-based diet. The results showed that she carries the DQ8 gene but was negative for antibodies. After the tests, even though they were negative and may have even been a false-negative due to her many other auto-immune conditions, she went on a paleo diet removing gluten completely in an effort to help heal her other auto-immune diseases. After six months of being completely gluten-free, she reintroduced gluten and got very sick. It turns out she is reactive to gluten. We will not know whether or not she has celiac disease unless she undergoes a biopsy while eating gluten. Not long after she gave up gluten, she realized she is also dairy intolerant.

My brother, the lover of artisan bread, finds that after a week of eating bread he gets sore joints but flat out refuses to get tested for celiac disease. He said, *"I can't live a life without wheat. I would rather get the joy from eating my bread, pastries, and pizza for as long as I can and die young, then give it up to live longer."* Some people just don't want to know.

Can you ever really heal from celiac disease?

In most cases, yes you can. But healing does not mean cured. You may heal your body, regenerate your intestines and live a healthy happy life, but the sad truth of it is, you won't be 'cured' of celiac disease no matter how long you eliminate gluten for. Celiac disease is for life. I only ever needed the one iron transfusion when I was diagnosed; it was enough to sustain me for a few months whilst my intestines regenerated and once they had, I was absorbing iron and nutrients from food like there was no tomorrow. The proof was in the regular blood tests to monitor my levels, and the weight that I started to gain. All of a sudden, I needed to exercise more than before, even though I wasn't eating more and probably eating better than ever.

But what if you don't heal?

When following a 100% gluten-free diet (GFD) and lifestyle, after a few months your villi should be well on its way to healing and after a couple of years, you should be living a healthy, happy lifestyle. A study at the Mayo Clinic looked at several hundred patients with follow up biopsies; after two years, it showed only 1/3 of the group recovered and after the five year mark, only two thirds.[51]

Sometimes, people think they are sticking to a 100% GFD but don't know that gluten is sneaking in. Low level gluten exposure through misunderstood ingredients and cross-contamination are thought to be one of the main reasons.

If significant problems persist there is a condition that's called refractory celiac disease (RCeD), which affects around 1.5% of celiac disease patients. It is a rare condition and comes with some very serious health complications because, essentially, you're at a greater risk of other degenerative diseases just like someone with undiagnosed celiac disease. If this is suspected, it may require a meeting with a dietician to help reboot a GFD and see if that helps. Failing that, there may be a need to swallow a camera to view the entire intestine to confirm the diagnosis. Further treatment is determined from there.

Quick recap

- Around 1% of most populations have celiac disease, yet most of them are undiagnosed. Around 20% of celiac disease patients do not experience any of the usual gastrointestinal upsets like sickness, bloating, rashes, etc. However, they can still be suffering from other complications.

- Undiagnosed celiac disease can be linked with cancer, diabetes, infertility, miscarriage, thyroid disease, multiple sclerosis, anemia, osteoporosis, epilepsy, and more.

---

[51] Rubio-Tapia, A., Rahim, M.W., See, J.A., Lahr, B.D., Wu, T.T., and Murray, J.A. (2010). "Mucosal recovery and mortality in adults with celiac disease after treatment with a gluten-free diet." Am J Gastroenterol, 105(6):1412-1420. doi:10.1038/ajg.2010.10

- Celiac disease is an auto-immune disease and once activated it can never be cured.

- Strictly adhering to a gluten-free diet is the only means to treat the disease. The symptoms will resolve with time, but the disease remains with you for life.

- If you eliminate gluten from your diet and regenerate your villi, it is extremely likely that you will absorb nutrients from food again and live a normal healthy life.

Chapter 10

The Bonnie & Clyde
of Your Guts

Have you ever heard of American couple Bonnie & Clyde who lived through the Great Depression? They were bank robbers, ran with their gang, and killed people along the way. They were not very nice people, to say the least.

You might think to yourself, "What the hell do they have to do with celiac disease?"

It's my simple analogy to explain to you two most significant and extremely unknown nasty elements that can cause harm to the body. Bonnie and Clyde are really called leaky gut and chronic inflammation.

These two rascals go hand-in-hand and can cause all sorts of damage to the body in areas you've never even thought about.

If you have celiac disease or are even just gluten intolerant, it's highly likely that you could be suffering from the damage of Bonnie & Clyde (leaky gut and chronic inflammation) as well. It's not all doom and gloom though. The good news is, if you heal one, the others will heal too.

Leaky gut

I hinted at the concept of leaky gut in the previous chapter. Let's look at this further.

Underneath your villi is a protective lining of cells that are joined together by *tight junctures*. In a healthy person, the villi are supposed to catch the nutrients from the chyme and pull it through this tightly junctured lining of your intestines and into your bloodstream. While they draw nutrients in, they also protect your body by keeping undigested food particles and toxins out. A gluten reaction, toxins, inflammation, stress, and a host of other issues can tear this cell wall making those tiny tight junctions bigger. Unnaturally bigger, so instead of looking like a cheese cloth, it looks like a tennis racket. This can allow gluten fractions to pass through the protective lining into your bloodstream and into your (inner) body. Not only can the gluten protein get in but also undigested food particles along with other nasty toxins that aren't supposed to. This is called leaky gut.

What is the Z-factor?

Z is for zonulin, an inflammatory protein that helps regulate the gut by opening and closing those tight junctures. Zonulin is triggered by harmful pathogens and one of the more powerful ones is gluten. This trigger occurs whether or not you're celiac, so even someone who is not celiac has their zonulin levels spike when gluten is eaten. It can open up the tight junctures and allow food particles and other toxins to get into the bloodstream. Anyone can have a leaky gut, not just celiacs. Gluten is not the only harmful pathogen that can stimulate zonulin. Bacteria is the other most powerful trigger, so even if you're gluten-free, you could still have your zonulin triggered by lurking bacteria.

This process of widening tight junctions and toxins entering the bloodstream is called leaky gut syndrome. It's more clinically known as *intestinal hyperpermeability*.

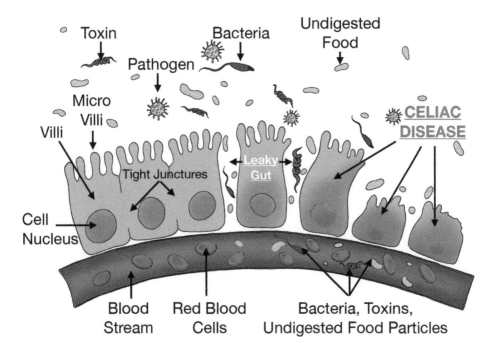

When these undigested particles and toxins get into your bloodstream, they are now officially inside your internal body. They are making their way around to various parts of your body through your bloodstream like a geek trolling the aisles at a Comic-Con convention! They can float through the bloodstream to many other parts of your body, from your brain to your toes. When they get there and stop they can cause inflammation which can lead to a whole host of issues.

A simple example is a bit of toxin, protein, or undigested food particle has flowed through your blood and landed in your knee joint. Your body says, *"Hey, there is something there that shouldn't be,"* so your immune system gathers up its soldiers to attack that foreign particle. Inflammation now occurs in the joint and prolonged inflammation leads to pain in the knee. Most people would think that they are getting old-age knees and would never think to attribute it to their gut.

When you have leaky gut, think about just how many toxins could make their way into your blood. Think of all the food you eat that has chemicals in it. Even toxic chemicals riding on your leafy unwashed salad may get in. The gluten protein may get in.

Does that mean that eating healthy food can cause leaky gut syndrome? Well, it depends on what you define as *healthy food*. Are you free from sugar, alcohol, medications, modified starches, processed food, additives, colorings, etc.? You're getting my drift here, right? These types of foods can be somewhat unavoidable, and bacteria can be unavoidable.

Once leaky gut has occurred, inflammation sets in anywhere it can.

Your liver is also at risk. Your liver is designed to filter the blood from your intestines, and right now it's in overdrive trying to sieve out all those toxins. But the job just gets too hard, too constant, and your liver is getting stressed out. This can lead to another wide variety of problems like liver inflammation and fatty liver disease. I don't think anyone wants to have a liver transplant, do they? Well, that's what happens when your liver shuts down.

You can present the same symptoms and reactions to these food particles in your bloodstream like you might to gluten. I hear of people continuously reporting they still feel sick when they changed to a gluten-free diet and one reason could be leaky gut. Just going gluten-free may not fix leaky gut and inflammation if you consume unhealthy gluten-free alternative food!

Symptoms of Leaky Gut		
Autism	Food Sensitives	Irritable Bowel Syndrome
Auto-Immune Disease	Gas/Bloating	Malabsorption
Brain Fog	Headaches	Mood Swings
Chronic Fatigue	Hormonal Imbalances	Nausea
Chron's Disease	Inflammatory Skin Conditions	Thyroid Problems

As you can see, some symptoms on this list present the same for celiac disease and gluten intolerance. Throw in a few others like targeted muscle spasms, bacteria overgrowth, and candida, and you have a hell of a lot to deal with on top of dealing with the gluten-related issues. Now you can see how the problems are mounting up on you faster than ever.

For some celiacs, there is a high probability that you have this leaky gut syndrome. They mostly go hand in hand, so unfortunately you can get a double dose of destruction.

It doesn't stop there. Your bloodstream also goes to your brain. Protecting your brain from what's allowed in is the blood/brain barrier. When those tiny junctures are widened (the cheese cloth turns into a tennis racket), bacteria and particles cross into your brain and you're now dealing with free radical damage to the brain. Just like the knee can get arthritic pain from inflammation, your brain can get inflamed. Where do you think your *brain fog* comes from? What about headaches and mood swings? This brain inflammation is called *neuroinflammation* and can be very serious.

Neuroinflammation left untreated becomes *chronic neuroinflammation*[52] which can lead to damage of the nervous system, Alzheimer's disease, Parkinson's disease, and Multiple Sclerosis!

Wow—this snowball just keeps going and going.

The biggest downside to leaky gut is that there aren't really any clinical tests that can be performed to achieve a proper diagnosis. The best way to find out if you have leaky gut is to assess all the symptoms you might have that correlate with leaky gut. Then follow an anti-inflammatory diet and monitor your symptoms for improvement. If you get better—then you probably had leaky gut. It's more common than you know.

So that, in a nutshell, is leaky gut and briefly described within that, is inflammation. Let's look at what inflammation is in more detail.

Inflammation

Inflammation can affect every part of the body, from your little pinky toe on your foot to the hair on the head, and it usually stems from the gut.

Acute inflammation is an inflammatory response to tissue injury and infection and is another protective mechanism in your body. Inflammation is not a bad thing in *small doses* when it can *do the job it's designed to.*

Have you ever sprained your ankle, and it blew up like a balloon? This is an *acute* inflammatory response to protect the joint. It swells around the area to mobilize and protect the joint while your body clears the dead cells and the tissue

---

[52] Chen W.W., Zhang, X., and Huang, W.J. (2016). "Role of neuroinflammation in neurodegenerative diseases (Review)." *Mol Med Rep., 13*(4):3391–3396. doi:10.3892/mmr.2016.4948

repairs. Once your cells have healed, the inflammation disappears, and life returns to normal.

This same process happens to your internal organs if they are acutely damaged, but sometimes the damage *isn't* always from an accident.

The other type of inflammation is called *chronic inflammation*[53] and it can be your worst nightmare because it can be silently fatal. Chronic inflammation is predominantly caused by diet and lifestyle. **This refers to coffee, alcohol, dairy, processed foods, sugar, fast food, stress, and lack of exercise.**

Chronic inflammation typically starts in the gut (as this is where you interact with the outside world) then it spreads to other parts of the body. This chronic inflammation is a silent killer! It can lead to many conditions that start affecting the body in different ways like cancer, auto-immune disease, and heart disease. But it can also lead to eyesight degradation, hair loss, and skin disorders, and it can manifest itself almost anywhere in the body, in any form.

So, the hamster wheel continues. You go back to the doctor who prescribes you drugs to treat your problem, which is *actually a symptom*, while never addressing the **underlying cause** of the problem which is inflammation. If you treat the inflammation by removing the cause, the problem will go away and not just that problem, but any other problems you may have too.

There are people who seek treatment for multiple forms of ailments such as diabetes, high blood pressure, fibromyalgia, and arthritis, and are taking multiple sets of drugs to treat each one of those issues, not knowing that inflammation may be the cause of them all.

Charlotte Gerson (the daughter of the famous Max Gerson who developed a dietary based alternative cancer treatment)[54] once said,

"You cannot heal selectively; you can't heal one disease and keep two others; it's impossible. When the body heals, IT HEALS."

Another example of a chronic inflammation-manifested disease is heart disease. Clogged arteries result in people having heart attacks! When inflammation occurs for heart disease patients, the endothelial cells that line the walls of the

[53] Pahwa, R., Goyal, A., Bansal, P., et al. (2020). Chronic Inflammation. StatPearls Publishing: Treasure Island, FL. Retrieved from: https://www.ncbi.nlm.nih.gov/books/NBK493173/
[54] College of Naturopathic Medicine. (Dec 11, 2012). "The Gerson Therapy - Charlotte Gerson on Cancer". YouTube, https://www.youtube.com/watch?v=quuvi6Gvvmc

arteries rupture. When this rupture occurs, the body releases plaque into the artery wall to lay down a barrier on the inside of the artery wall to plug the holes. Kind of like putting a bandage over a wound.

However, if the *source* of the inflammation that *caused* the rupture does not go away, more and more ruptures occur. The body keeps putting layer upon layer of bandages down until they get so thick that they clog the artery. Once the artery is fully clogged, a heart attack can occur which is usually fatal! Often, the first symptom of heart disease *is* death. Only the lucky ones will be forewarned with angina pains, and many of these are mostly mistaken for muscle pains in the shoulder, neck, jaw, or back.

What is the medical treatment for heart disease? Bypass surgery and lots of drugs with negative side effects. What happens when you don't remove the cause (inflammation) of the disease? Another clogged artery, a lifelong commitment to drugs, or death. Many people have had more than one by-pass operation because they do not remove the cause of the inflammation.

Why is dairy on the list of items that can cause inflammation?

Dairy can cause inflammation through mucus build up in the stomach. People can also be susceptible to hidden food allergies in dairy such as lactose (sugar compound) or casein (protein), which can also lead to a host of other physical and neurological problems. Dairy consumption may also increase the acid levels in the body. I'm sure you've heard of a pH balance before. It is used in many applications, and it is the balance between acid and alkaline. Dairy consumption can tip the scales to the acidic side, which is *not* really a good thing.

Now, I'm not advocating you eliminate dairy from your diet; you have to work that one out for yourself. What I do advocate is listen to your body, understand the real science behind dairy consumption and what it does, and adjust your diet according to what works for you. A study in Italy uncovered that 24 percent of patients who had a dairy intolerance also had celiac disease.[55]

After I had eliminated gluten, I noticed that I got a clogged nose with mucus when I ate dairy. This was probably happening before I went gluten-free, but I did

---

[55] Ojetti, V., Nucera, G., Migneco, A., Gabrielli, M., Lauritano, C., Danese, S., Assunta Zocco, M. Nista, E., Cammarota, G., de Lorenzo, A., Gasbarrini, G., and Gasbarrini, A. (2005). "High Prevalence of Celiac Disease in Patients with Lactose Intolerance". Digestion, 71:106-110. doi: 10.1159/000084526

not realize it. So, I went to the Facebook forums to see who else in the world might have had a similar thing happen and again, the response was astounding. I would say that well over half of the people I spoke to with celiac disease were also dairy intolerant! There are dedicated Facebook groups set up purely for the gluten *and* dairy intolerant.

For me, that means I don't drink milk unless necessary (there are great alternatives like almond and coconut milk), but I do eat cheese on occasion as I just can't go without a creamy French brie with my vintage Italian Shiraz, or a good Mexican queso dip and corn chips. I try to have a balance of being good 90% of the time. If I have to put up with a snotty nose and a little rumble in the jungle every so often so I can enjoy life, I will. My husband, however, has a different view of the situation as he is usually the one who is *dutch-ovened* in the middle of the night from a fermented brie cheese fart gone sour!

I know this list is a little daunting: *coffee, alcohol, dairy, processed foods, sugar, fast food.* Most of us are exposed to these elements daily, and the thought of cutting some of it out really sucks. Inflammation isn't just restricted to diet; it is also caused by lifestyle factors such as stress, lack of sleep, and lack of exercise.

Inflammation can accelerate the body's aging process inside and out, which leads to the degradation of the body's cells, including the collagen in the skin and the elasticity in the connective tissues. That's not so nice for us women who want to stay looking young and youthful. We spend so much money on topical creams, facials, and other beauty related products but that's all on the surface and is mostly a waste of time and money if you don't start from the inside by cooling the inflammation and soothing the gut.

How on-going chronic inflammation and celiac disease are linked

Many people will swap directly to gluten-free alternative products. Instead of wheat pasta, they will eat corn pasta. Instead of wheat bread, they will eat gluten-free bread that's made up of 20 different chemicals and modified starches. So, the problem is, although you may think you are healing from celiac disease by removing gluten from your diet, if you are not careful with what alternative products you eat, you could be causing on-going and chronic inflammation in the body. This is one of the biggest and most important lessons I've learned about this gluten-free lifestyle that I want to share with you. I believe it's one of the most lesser known yet most significant issues that plague many of us. As I've mentioned before, many people with celiac disease have many other conditions and issues going on, and I believe inflammation is the key factor that's linking them together.

How can we reduce inflammation?

- Simply think, *what does it mean to be healthy?* and you will have some answers. If you consume any of the inflammatory factors listed above, perhaps review how much you consume and try a little less.
- Try adding in some exercise to your day.
- Getting quality sleep is vital.
- Power up with some supplements to support your diet is another great way.

But don't forget the family of trillions you have living inside you, they too need to be taken care of. By supporting our gut to have a healthy population of bacteria, they can help reduce inflammation to the immune system[56] so it can work properly to protect you when needed; support the digestive system so you process food properly; and help your overall body. You can support your little itty-bitty critters by feeding them a good diet of food, and taking probiotics as a supplement.

Think carefully before buying a packaged food item. See if there is a better quality brand or product or even if you can make the product yourself from scratch.

For me, I know that coffee causes inflammation, but I'm aware of it and only have one cup in the morning to feed my brain addiction. There have been some reported health benefits to drinking coffee. Whether or not they are true, I can't say, but I won't use this as a reason to drink four cups a day. I love my wine and understand it also causes inflammation, so I try to have wine only two nights a week. You still need to live life and find a balance. If anyone can go without these items altogether then my hat's off to you.

A personal story: how I learned inflammation and diet are important

I mentioned earlier in **My Rant & Rave** chapter that my father had heart disease. Well, luckily enough, he didn't die of his heart attack! When he was at the hospital having an angiogram[57] they found he had one fully clogged and two 50%

---

[56] Plaza-Díaz, J., Ruiz-Ojeda, F.J., Vilchez-Padial, L.M., and Gil, A. (2017). "Evidence of the Anti-Inflammatory Effects of Probiotics and Synbiotics in Intestinal Chronic Diseases". Nutrients, 9(6):555. doi:10.3390/nu9060555

[57] A dye is injected into the bloodstream to reveal clogged arteries.

clogged arteries and wanted to schedule him for a triple bypass immediately. The human body is amazing at survival and the only reason my father was still alive is that he grew a vein from the left side of his heart to his right to keep feeding it some blood. The stubborn old bastard grew a new artery! Small as it was, it was that millimeter-wide tube that kept him alive. We couldn't believe his luck.

My father grew up as a farmer, then turned builder for most of his adult life. He lived off of bacon and eggs, white bread, cookies, chocolate, beer, coffee, milk, and drank a 1.5-litre Coke every day. He ate meat every single day and for most of his meals. He never ate salad, calling it *rabbit food*. His was a classic case that, over many years, was causing ongoing, chronic inflammation to his body through diet. Exercise wasn't a problem because he was physically active all day long, and he was not overweight; he had an ok body for his age. He wasn't even 60.

Despite my pleas and cries, he flat out refused to have any surgery and was willing to die before going onto a surgeon's table. *Stubborn old bastard*, I thought. How is this logic for you? He said to me that there was a 3% chance he would die on the table, so he didn't want to go through with the surgery. My response was, "*You silly old man, you'll die if you don't!*" But he dug his heels in and walked out of the hospital, one slow, painful step at a time. He refused to take the copious amounts of drugs prescribed to him, too.

Infuriated as I was, I cut a deal with him. If he didn't have surgery, he had to do everything the natural way and *my* way—no ifs, ands, or buts allowed. Reluctantly, he agreed.

Guess what we did first? We removed all the causes of inflammation I could find. I put him on a juice/vegan food diet. No sugar, no alcohol, no coffee, and no meat. Nothing but leafy green rabbit food, vegetables, fresh fruit, and a ton of supplements. We found a natural solution for the blood-thinning drug they wanted him to take and that was raw garlic. We found a natural solution for blood pressure statin drugs and that was Ubiquinol.[58]

I took him to a German functional medicine doctor (PhD) who specialized in treating cancer patients without the use of chemo and drugs. I took my father every week to have two liters of vitamin therapy and chelation therapy administered through an IV drip. Chelation is a solution that binds to heavy metals and calcium

---

[58] An advanced form of the nutrient Coenzyme Q10, a vitamin-like substance made naturally in the body

in the blood to help flush arteries out. The vitamins were a mixture of vitamin C and various others to flood the body with nutrients and antioxidants.

The IV therapy continued for six months and when that concluded, my dad continued to maintain the new vegan diet. Around the 12-month mark, we re-introduced grass-fed cuts of meat and other little treats. I remember the look on his face when he ate his first lamb chop in a year. It was priceless.

When we started, my father could not walk 10 feet without having severe angina pain. Now, he is back on a building site every day, working just like he used to. His clogged arteries naturally cleared themselves enough for blood to flow more freely and along with the help of his newly grown artery, he now enjoys a very happy, healthy, and fit lifestyle, and the occasional beer.

This is just an example of how the body can heal when you remove the root cause of the problem and in this instance, the cause was INFLAMMATION! I've heard of many people having multiple bypass operations in their lifetime, simply because after surgery they return to the lifestyle they had beforehand and they do not improve.

My father's diagnosis occurred several years before I was diagnosed with celiac disease. I was no expert on the matter but having studied health and nutrition prior to his situation gave me the basis to study further into heart disease and learn all about inflammation. He became my test subject and I crash-coursed myself on the subject in my best effort to prevent him from kicking the bucket. Through his journey, I feel so very grateful to have had the time to learn about the effects of inflammation, learn from a PhD physician, and watch real-life changes actually work and become real-time solutions to what is such a significant problem that affects so many. It was at this point that I really realized what you eat can literally mean life or death.

Chapter 11

Just Because It Says
Gluten-Free
Doesn't Mean It's Good for You

So, you've been told you have celiac disease or you've discovered that you're gluten-intolerant and you think everything will be ok if you just go on a full gluten-free diet right? WRONG!!!!!

People following a 100% strict GF diet may still have:

- chronic inflammation

- poor vitamin status

- degradation of the villi due to cross contamination or lack of proper knowledge where gluten is present, and therefore are not on a 100% GFD

- a risk of developing other diseases

Understanding now how inflammation works, you could probably identify many other elements in your diet that are causing inflammation. Would you believe many of your gluten-free alternative products can cause inflammation? There are tons of companies cashing in on the *gluten-free* and *free-from* saga. To the uneducated individual, they remove the gluten but add in other inflammatory substances. Not only is it a cost to your wallet, it's a cost to your health.

Why do companies do this? Well, perhaps it's all about the dollar. If companies can make a product cheaper, faster, and still meet regulations, they probably will regardless of its diminishing nutritional benefits. You need to buy your products from reputable sources and in most cases, smaller, more independent companies who actually understand your condition and have a real passion for creating healthy alternatives.

After I got over the depression and hatred for this disease, I started to accept that there were alternatives out there that I could eat and I needed to start exploring this. I'd never eaten GF-alternative food before and had never even looked at any of the packaging, so when I saw my first loaf of GF bread, I was horrified!

I remember standing in the grocery store and I spotted a loaf of yummy-looking GF bread. I picked it up and began to walk towards the checkout with it when I thought to myself, *I better look at what's in this.*

I turned the packet over and noticed a few things. For a start, it was a chemical shit storm with the main ingredient being water, followed by *modified tapioca starch (E1442)*. Wanting to find out more about this prominent additive, I whipped out my iPhone with its unique E-Number application on it. I looked up E1442 and this was the result:

Hydroxypropyl Distarch Phosphate (E1442): a modified starch with risks to the digestive system and gluten intolerant people. Its purpose is a thickening and bulking agent.

This got my attention. Risks to the digestive system? Risks to gluten-intolerant people?

I stood there for a good 20 minutes Googling this additive and the more I found out about it, the more my jaw dropped.

So, this is how the monopolies in the food industry were able to start cashing in on the gluten-free movement. They remove the gluten to say *gluten-free* but put in what appears to be a toxic additive! This additive does not set off your immune response like gluten does, but it can cause inflammation.

This bread contained three other toxic-looking additives along with soy and maize (corn) starch. Needless to say, I put the bread back. I moved to the next loaf of GF bread and the same thing applied. Then the next, and the next, and sure enough, in this supermarket I was not able to buy a loaf of healthy, additive-free bread at all.

My excitement and motivation to try my first loaf of GF bread was utterly deflated, and I was upset that I was so close to consuming food that was going to keep me sick. This modified starch was not the only culprit in the gluten-free food products. Processed sugars, bad fats, corn, and soy were significantly present. Wheat flour seemed to be mostly replaced with refined starches from rice, corn, potato, and tapioca.

I knew then and there that I was not going to be able to live a long and healthy life by making a simple diet switch to gluten-free food. I *had* to delve deeper into this situation and blow the whistle. I needed to get educated. Understanding the diet in which I am forced to live was crucial so I could be in control of my life and my disease. Finding food, finding resources, and a community were key to making this shitty diagnosis a little less shitty.

This was a defining moment, a turning point in my life, and why I eventually created this book. As I learned about gluten-free diets and celiac disease, I combined it with my existing knowledge on inflammation. I thought I'd be able to help others avoid the trap of the gluten-free diet myth.

In the coming pages we will:

- learn about the 'big 3' ingredients added to gluten-free food

- identify harmful additives

- learn about how starches in GF foods affect the body

- get label savvy

- understand cross contamination and what it means for you

- learn about what healthy alternative product looks like

Number 1 of the 'big 3' - Sugar

Mmmmmm. Suuuugggggaaaarrrr…

I hear the TV character Homer Simpson saying this while drool leaks out the side of his mouth.

It's sweet, white, and looks very pretty on cakes. I recall in my younger years my mother putting sugar on so much of our food. We had a desert called *Banana, Sugar, & Cream* which was literally just that: a bowl full of chopped bananas followed by a cup of cream and a few tablespoons of sugar over the top. It was devilishly delicious and the memory of spending those after-dinner moments with my family was a treat in itself. Or I would see those beautiful gluten-filled apple turnovers coming out of the oven then served up with powdered sugar dusted over the top like snow. My grandmother would pick fresh strawberries from her garden, chop them up, and toss them in sugar. I have many wonderful memories around sugar even though I don't really have a sweet tooth. Sugar just takes me back to those happy memories.

But…

If you don't know by now that sugar in its refined form, even in small amounts, is bad for you, then you're in serious trouble. It can cause obesity,[59] addiction, disease,[60] and it can have an impact on the development of cancer.[61] Overall, it can cause inflammation.

I'm sure at some point in your life you've heard of *fat-free* marketing campaigns. This was and still is the biggest lie in history. It fooled so many people, my mother being one of them. She was addicted to buying products labeled fat-free, thinking they were healthier for her. I remember being in the shopping center with her and she would buy the yogurt tub that said 99% fat-free on it. Yes, it may be 99 % fat-free, but it contained far greater amounts of sugar than any other brand as a substitute for taste, which is worse!

It seems that marketing agencies and food companies around the globe jumped on the back of that stupid Ancel Keys publication[62] that touted FAT as the enemy. Companies appeared to join the movement in droves, creating 99% and 100% fat-free products, all the while boosting them with seriously large amounts of sugar. It makes marketing sense doesn't it? Plaster an inviting-looking label across the product saying fat-free to trick the consumer into thinking it's healthy for them, all the while hooking them with refined sugar for taste that will have them coming back for more. Over recent years Ancel Keys' publication has been debunked, and

---

[59] Johnson, R.J., Sánchez-Lozada, L.G., Andrews, P., Lanaspa, M.A.. (2017). "Perspective: A Historical and Scientific Perspective of Sugar and Its Relation with Obesity and Diabetes". Adv Nutr., 8(3):412-422. doi:10.3945/an.116.014654

[60] Freeman, C.R., Zehra, A., Ramirez, V., Wiers, C.E., Volkow, N.D., and Wang, G.J. (2018). "Impact of sugar on the body, brain, and behavior." Front Biosci (Landmark Ed), 23:2255-2266. Retrieved from: https://www.ncbi.nlm.nih.gov/pubmed/29772560

[61] Jiang, Y., Pan, Y., Rhea, P.R. et al. (2016). "A Sucrose-Enriched Diet Promotes Tumorigenesis in Mammary Gland in Part through the 12-Lipoxygenase Pathway." *Cancer Res.*, 76(1):24–29. doi:10.1158/0008-5472.CAN-14-3432

[62] Keys, A. et al. (1966). "Epidemiological studies related to coronary heart disease: Characteristics of men aged 40-59 in seven countries". *Acta Med Scand, 460:1-392.*

coincidentally companies are using the fat-free marketing triggers less nowadays. Now the tables have turned, and we have learned that fat is our friend and sugar is our enemy.

There are varying types of sugar to be aware of and each carry their own set of health risks.

- Fructose— from fruits

- Lactose—from milk

- Sucrose—refined sugar from cane

- High Fructose Corn Syrup—from corn

Fructose

When you eat fruit, the naturally occurring fructose is converted in the body to glucose to be used by every cell and transported to the brain. A natural process. Think back to the hunter-gatherer days; those hairy Neanderthals probably didn't have diabetes from eating fruit from trees. Fructose doesn't require insulin secreted from the pancreas to balance your blood sugar levels like what's needed when sucrose is ingested.

When the whole fruit is eaten, you are eating the fructose along with the fiber, which slows down the digestion and does not cause a spike in blood sugar levels. Fruit is amazingly nutritious, but it has been pillaged by the food industry and is now being used as an additive in packaged foods and drinks. When natural ingredients are converted into additives, they typically are no longer nutritious and, in some cases, can cause inflammation.

Lactose

Oh, the wonders of milk. Lactose is also a naturally occurring sugar compound found in milk. Not only in the milk of cows and other animals, but in human mother's milk as well. It provides essential life-giving nutrients to a newborn. However, every other species is weaned off milk eventually except humans. Why not humans? For some reason, it's become normal in our society to wean a baby off mother's milk but then substitute cow's milk for the rest of its life. I find this very odd considering a female cow weighs on average 730kg (1600 lbs) and has the protein, sugar, and enzymes in their milk to nourish a calf which weighs on average 136kg (300 lbs). Not a little baby that weighs 2kg. So, essentially, we are pumping babies full of lactose in the concentrations meant for a calf 10 times its size. Why not give steroids to a child?

Don't get me wrong, I also grew up on cow's milk. I had raw milk straight from the cow on our farm to drink and I am not telling anyone to consume or not consume it; that's up to the individual to work out. But perhaps when we are equipped with better knowledge we can make different educated choices. Don't forget this is all about listening and learning what is working and what is *not* working with our bodies.

Have you ever noticed that babies on formula derived from cow's milk are bigger and fatter than the average baby fed on mother's milk? I noticed this for myself when talking to friends who have kids. Then, after a few Google searches, I found the internet is littered with reports and articles validating my thoughts. I don't suppose the higher concentrations of lactose and protein would have something to do with it?

Why is it so ingrained in us to drink cow's milk? I read an interesting statement and that was over 65% of the world's population appears to have a reduced ability to digest lactose after infancy[63], yet it's one of the most globally consumed food sources. Surprise, surprise!

Many people who are gluten-intolerant or celiac also find themselves reacting to dairy. Dairy can cause an overabundance of mucus production in the gut. It's also an allergen and can cause inflammation. I also notice a build-up of mucus in my nose when I eat dairy, yet I never noticed it before until I removed other inflammatory factors from my diet. I couldn't see the forest for the trees. Not only can dairy cause inflammation, but lactose is used as an additive in many packaged products and especially gluten-free products. So, one who is not label savvy, may be avoiding lactose in mainstream dairy products but have not realized the rice crackers they just ate contains it.

Like meat, milk can come from very large production farms, so typically, the cow is pumped with growth hormones, antibiotics, and who knows what else to keep up with the demand for increased milk production. Can these hormones and antibiotics trickle down into the milk itself that you consume?

---

[63] Genetics Home Reference. (2010). "Lactose intolerance". Retrieved from: https://ghr.nlm.nih.gov/condition/lactose-intolerance#definition

Milk typically undergoes homogenization, meaning the fat is emulsified into the liquid so it does not separate, and then it undergoes a process of pasteurization, which is to sterilize the crap out of it so that those hormones, bacteria, and antibiotics are rendered harmless. But is this always the case? What we are left with, at that point, is white water that's full of sugar. One cup of milk contains 2.5 teaspoons of (lactose) sugar!

Sucrose

Ah, here we arrive to that wonderful white sweetness that delighted my gluten-laden deserts when I was a child. Before you picture those amazing cupcakes with icing sugar on top or that apple turnover, picture diabetes, a wrinkly face, and a fat dimpled ass instead!

Sucrose comes from those wonderful glistening cane stalks grown in the tropical climates that grace most of North Eastern Australia, Florida, Hawaii, and Louisiana. Typically, pure sugar cane juice that is pressed right out of the stalk has little effect on blood sugar levels, tastes amazing, and has health *benefits*. However, like all things processed and refined, sucrose is bad, bad, bad.

Sucrose and diabetes

When you eat a chocolate bar or a lollipop, sugar gets into your bloodstream quite quickly and you might feel your energy pick up. It's obvious in children as they run around like headless chickens. However, during that process your body says, *"Shit, there is too much sugar in the blood! Let's tell the pancreas to release insulin to grab hold of that sugar and store it in the muscles for use as energy down the road."*

Storing energy for later is not such a bad idea. It's a wonderful primal design *but* you probably ate that candy bar while sitting on your butt at work, and by the time you get home, it's dark and you don't feel like exercising and using up that stored energy. Flip forward to the next day and the same thing happens, and then the next. Your body then decides that there's no need for that energy to be stored in the muscles anymore and turns it into that yucky, jelly-like dimply substance on your ass. However, it's not just your ass that the fatty substance is deposited to; it gets put all around your *organs*! This is called visceral fat.

Have you ever felt tired about an hour after eating something sugary? Or have you seen kids run around like crazy then just hit the deck and sleep like a log?

That's what happens when the insulin has done its job; your blood sugar level has dropped and you don't feel that energy rush anymore. There is no more sugary blood feeding the brain.

It's very easy for this to happen as starches and modified starches produce a similar result to sucrose. Throughout the day, your blood sugar levels go up-down-up-down-up-down like a rollercoaster because of the average diet.

Breakfast = bagel & cream cheese

Lunch = ham & salad baguette

Afternoon snack = muesli/snack bar/Mars Bar™

Dinner = pasta

But now *years* have passed and your poor pancreas finally gives in and says, *"I can't do my job anymore. You've broken me."* Your blood sugar levels get dangerously high, stay there, and you can end up with type II diabetes.

Sugar just doesn't make you fat; it can make you age quicker too!

All forms of processed sugar can make your skin sag, age, and lines and wrinkles form where you don't want them. Sugar goes on the hunt in the body to bind itself with proteins, forming a new sugar-protein substance called AGE (Advanced Glycation End-Product). How coincidental the acronym. Before you know it, you're only 40 and you're getting your first grey hair!

High fructose corn syrup (HFCS)

Oh, the wonders of agriculture. Who would have thought you could take the juicy corn kernel from the cob and turn it into a highly refined artificial sweetener? This is HFCS, and it's the devil in disguise. This refined sweetener is worse for you than table sugar, converts to fat more quickly in the body than sugar, and is currently under investigation for being one of the leading causes of obesity in the United States. HFCS makes a bee-line straight to your liver and switches on fat production, resulting in fatty-liver diseases. It's so cheap to produce that it's added to so many gluten-free foods it's crazy. Also, to add a double whammy into the mix, the corn used is typically GMO corn!

Common Foods that Contain HFCS		
Biscuits	Coffee Creamer	Jam/Jelly
Bread	Energy Drinks	Salad Dressing
Boxed Dinners	Frozen Snack Food	Sauces & Condiments
Candy	Granola Bars	Soda Pop
Canned Fruit Juice	Ice Cream	Yoghurt

HFCS also gets disguised with other names, making it all the more confusing to find. Here are some other names to watch:

- natural corn syrup

- isolated fructose

- maize syrup

- glucose/fructose syrup

Overall, sugar is pro-inflammatory and not ideal to be over-consumed when trying to heal the body.

Tying it all together

Sugar in these various forms weasel their way into so many gluten-free products. Much like the fat-free marketing campaign was able to trick consumers into thinking they were making a healthier choice, gluten-free seems to be marketed in a similar way. To the uneducated, picking up a product because it says gluten-free in effort to make a better choice might in fact land you a product that contains a significant amount of refined or highly processed sugar instead. Avoiding gluten is one thing, but it would be also good for you to start learning how these exceptionally pro-inflammatory additives will or will not make their way into your new diet. This is the first of '*the big 3*' in gluten-free food.

Here is a little quotation that resonated with me because it's short and easily remembered. Hopefully, it will resonate with you too.

Sugar makes you fat...Fat gives you energy!

Number 2 of 'the big 3' - The great soy debate

Ah, soy. I find I have a love/hate relationship with soy. On one hand, soy used in ancient Asian cultures was an excellent source of protein. On the other hand, it's used widely as a terrible additive in so many western food products.

Soy, or soya bean, is a legume native to East Asia. The people in Okinawa Japan who consume soy can live healthily to over 100 years old. However, the soy *they* consume differs vastly from the type *we* consume daily. This little beast hides like gluten in so many foods.

Soy, in its **unfermented state**, can wreak havoc on the body. It can disrupt the hormone system, block the absorption of magnesium and calcium, cause gastric distress, and mimic estrogen in the body, which is bad for both men and women.

You will typically see unfermented soy in items such as soy milk, tofu, edamame and alternative vegetarian foods.

Guess who is the largest producer of soy in the world? You might think Asia as that's where it originated but guess again. It's the United States![64]

The *agricultural industries* who manufacture soya bean crops (notice how I say *manufacture* and not *grow*) have published tons of articles and so-called research data on the health benefits of soy. In my opinion, I think it's mostly bullshit and you will see why below for yourself.

Soy is the second largest crop manufactured in the USA after corn.

That wonderful weed killer we use in the gardens called RoundUp™ is also the weed-killer used on most of the soy crops throughout the United States. The active ingredient in RoundUp™ is called glyphosate and was patented in the 1970s by Monsanto. In the mid-1990s, Monsanto released the first RoundUp Ready® genetically modified beans which are glyphosate-resistant. These soybeans can be sprayed with RoundUp™ throughout their growing life and not die! To give you an idea of how powerful this product is, RoundUp™ says on their website to kill a mature tree you need to drill holes into the trunk and inject it with 1ml of undiluted solution. Even if you did 10 holes, that's only two teaspoons of

---

[64] Karuga, J. (2018). "10 Countries With Largest Soybean Production". World Atlas. Retrieved from: https://www.worldatlas.com/articles/world-leaders-in-soya-soybean-production-by-country.html

RoundUp™ to kill an entire tree! Can you imagine how much of this stuff is sprayed on the soybeans?

Big Agriculture has managed to separate the soy protein and soy oil from the humble bean and now soybean oil accounts for 90% of the USA's oil production according to the USDA. Soy oil and soy-derived additives have weaseled their way into all sorts of food products from baby formula to potato chips. They even show up in cosmetics, nutritional supplements, crayons, adhesives, and even animal feed.

Many packaged foods and especially gluten-free alternatives contain soy derivatives. Would it baffle you to think that crumbed fish and chips can contain soy oil? Or what about rice crackers? These are seemingly unrelated products that one might not think would use soy derivatives. Just like wheat, HFCS, and hydrogenated oils, soy also is disguised with many different names.

I said at the start of the chapter that you and I are consuming it daily, now you know how. It's used widely in packaged products and comes in many different names. Avoiding products containing soy isn't just as easy as ditching tofu and soy sauce. Soy is in just as many products as gluten.

Other names that may mean Soy ingredients		
Artificial Flavour	Hydrolysed Vegetable Protein	Mono-diglyceride
Glycine Max	Kinako	Natural Flavouring
Hydrolysed Soy Protein	Lecithin	Textured Vegetable Protein

Common Products Containing Soy		
Biscuits	Margarine	Soybean Oil
Chocolate	Mayonnaise	Soy Flour
Crackers	Pastries	Soy Milk
Lecithin	Potato Chips / Crisps	Tofu

Even though Australia and the UK may not grow soy crops like the USA, that doesn't mean GMO soy is not being used in your imported products. Luckily, soy is listed as an allergen in the United States and Australia, so if you want to avoid products containing soy and are not sure how to spot technical names, look for it listed as an allergen.

Eating food products that contain soy-derivatives not only wreaks havoc on the body in so many ways but can kill off the good bacteria in your gut and can damage your digestive system. This is what you are working hard to protect right now.

The consumption of soy in an unfermented state has been linked to a multitude of health problems along with causing inflammation.

Unfermented Soy Consumption Related Disorders		
Brain Damage	Food Allergies	Infertility
Breast Cancer	Heart Disease	Leaky Gut
Cognitive Problems	Immune System Impairment	Ovarian Cancer
Digestive Difficulty	Infant Abnormalities	Thyroid Disorders

Remember that nasty anti-nutrient I talked about earlier called lectin? The one that causes inflammation and damage to the body? Well, soya beans contain some of the highest amounts of lectin   .

Asians have been eating soy for thousands of years without problem, including those long-living Okinawans, so how come they don't have the same health issues we have?

The simple answer is their soy is a natural, non-GMO, homegrown soy that is *fermented* using ancient techniques. Natto is the type of soy consumed in Okinawa where age expectancy is extremely high. Put simply, they aren't eating frozen crumbed fish and chips, potato chips, and lollies (candy) with GMO unfermented hydrogenated soya bean oil in it.

Fermenting the soya bean makes the bean digestion friendly. They are rich in probiotics and have a high source of vitamin K2 which helps build strong bones, supports brain health, and aids in healing the body.

Another example of fermented soy is miso paste, and I'm sure at one point you've tried a delicious warm miso soup. If you haven't, then you're missing out. But then again, not all miso soups are created equal either. The instant version you may have seen at your local grocery store is full of additives that can be harmful to the body. I purchase my miso paste from a reputable organic supplier through my health food store in the form of a pure stone ground paste.

Soy sauce, one of the most common staples in Asian cuisine, is one of the world's oldest condiments, dating back 2,500 years from China. It was made from collecting the drippings of miso (fermented soybean paste) and mixing it with water and salt. In this time-honored tradition, this fermentation process also neutralizes the unhealthy component of the soybean. Today, soy sauce manufacturing is on such a large scale that most manufacturers utilize a chemical process known as acid hydrolysis and do not use a fermentation process. Many commercial companies use **wheat** to make their soy sauce. It's cheaper for the consumer and does the same job. This can make eating out at Asian restaurants challenging. However, there are alternatives.

I recommend tamari, the Japanese version of soy sauce. It's thicker in consistency, less salty, and in most cases, follows the old ways of fermentation and production. The brand I buy is fermented for six months.

If you want to go completely soy-free and are not keen on tamari, then check out Bragg's® Organic Coconut Aminos. It's a natural and organic soy-free option and made from non-GMO organic coconut nectar, sea salt, distilled water, and organic apple cider vinegar. It is a great replacement for soy sauce, tamari, Worcestershire, etc. I love using this for my cauliflower fried rice dishes. It contains a wide variety of minerals, vitamin C, Bs, and 17 amino acids.

So, now you know what the great soy debate is all about. The take-away tips are:

- Do not consume generic soy sauce that contains wheat

- Use a gluten-free soy sauce, or better still tamari when cooking at home

- Stay clear of vegetarian products that contain soy like soy sausages, burger patties, etc.

- Avoid unfermented products like edamame and be mindful of cheap miso soups

- If you like tofu, try to find a traditional version that's fermented or swap to tempeh

- Keep an eye out for soy ingredients on the back of packaged food. In most instances, it will list soy in the allergen section of the label. Put it back and find an alternative if you can

Overall, just be mindful when making purchases as gluten-free products can contain quite a large amount of soy and other nasties that can do you harm. Just because it says gluten-free doesn't mean it's healthy for you. But don't despair, this is all part of the learning process.

When you're at the shops, or even shopping online and you find a packet of crackers and it says it contains soy, just take the time to find one that doesn't. You can practically buy anything you want without soy, you just have to find it first. Once you have gone through this process a few times, you will start to develop your usual go-to products and shopping will become easier.

You don't need to avoid soy like the plague or let this information overwhelm you, as you already have enough to deal with trying to avoid gluten but making better educated choices all forms part of leading a healthy and happy life.

Number 3 of 'the big 3' - King corn

What is all the buzz, fuss, and confusion surrounding corn?

Corn has been around for as long as I can remember and is a staple part of any diet, right? What about eating fresh hot corn on the cob with butter? What about popcorn at the movies? What about those juicy yellow corn kernels as a side dish to a roast? Corn chips and salsa anyone?

Surely it can't be that bad?

Corn originated around 9,000 years ago in Central America at the start of the agricultural shift in history. But corn back then looked nothing like the corn we see today. Original corn was tiny, around 2-3 centimeters in length, and had only 5 to 10 very hard small kernels. These kernels needed to be broken open by hammering them with a hard object. They were dry and tasted like a raw potato. There were approximately eight known varieties of corn back then.

Today, corn is grown in 69 countries with an annual production of 790 million tons. The USA is the largest producer in the world[65] as of 2020. Corn today is 20-30 centimeters long and contains hundreds of kernels. It's super easy to peel, steams in minutes, and tastes sweet and juicy.

Like soy and wheat, corn has been twisted, turned, shaped, extracted, and mixed with a multitude of chemicals to turn the simple corn kernel into a ton of other additives used in food production today. Nearly all of these *corn alternatives* are inflammatory to the body.

What happened and when did it all change?

Over thousands of years, the humble original corn from Central America had the very best kernels picked and replanted to create stronger yielding crops. Repeat the process over generations and just like with wheat, corn began to change.

Enter the industrial food revolution where food is now being produced on a massive scale, including corn. The USA exploded in production and corn became one of the easiest and most lucrative crops for farmers to grow. In the 1950s the average bushel of corn per acre was 39; today, it sits somewhere around 180 to 200!

> Corn is the second most genetically modified food on the planet after soy.

Like soy, corn has been bred to withstand glyphosate, the toxic weed killer. It's practically impossible to buy non-GMO corn anymore in the USA. Luckily, Australia and some other countries do not produce GMO corn. However, how can you be certain of what you're buying in a packet of pasta? Let's say that pasta is made in Italy but the corn flour they are using is imported from the United States. You can be pretty certain it's GMO corn flour. While the USA is the largest producer of corn in the world, around 20% is exported to other countries.

What about your other imported products like corn chips, crackers, biscuits, sauces, and gravy mixes? How can you be certain they are not made from GMO ingredients?

When buying gluten-free products, corn and soy are commonly used as additives.

---

[65] Shahbandeh, M. (2020)."Corn production by country 2018/2019". Retrieved from: https://www.statista.com/statistics/254292/global-corn-production-by-country/

Here are a few examples of corn additives; some of them have confusing names.

Other Names for Corn Additives		
Citric Acid	Dextrin	Malt
Confections Sugar	Dextrose	Mono & Diglycerides
Corn Flour	Fructose	Monosodium Glutamate
Corn Fructose	Lactic Acid	Sorbitol

So, how does the change in corn production and these corn derivatives affect us today?

Corn is a pro-inflammatory food! Meaning it can cause inflammation in the body when eaten. The same applies for the derivatives of corn. Corn contains a protein that is difficult to digest like gluten. It's high in calories and low in nutrients. Corn can cause inflammation for everyone; however, for celiacs it has become quite a concern.

Many gluten intolerant/celiac patients report the same physical effects to corn as they have with eating gluten. Although corn does not initiate the same auto-immune response as gluten, celiacs may be experiencing the damage from the inflammation. It could be upsetting leaky gut syndrome and they could be reacting to the lectins.

Grain and corn are also used as food sources for animals. So, if you buy a cheap cut of meat from a supermarket, it could be from a cow that's fed in a factory farm with wheat and corn its whole life. So far, there have been links[66] from grain-fed meat to inflammatory conditions such as heart disease, diabetes, cancer, and obesity.

Corn can be hard to avoid. Corn is widely used in gluten-free products as a direct additive; it's in many pastas, flours, and packaged foods. It also does not fall

[66] Provenza, F. D., Kronberg, S. L., and Gregorini, P. (2019). "Is Grassfed Meat and Dairy Better for Human and Environmental Health?". Frontiers in nutrition, 6, 26. https://doi.org/10.3389/fnut.2019.00026/

under any of the allergens for labeling so trying to keep an eye out for all the technical names that look nothing like corn can be a daunting task.

What's the takeaway?

- Avoid corn derived additives in gluten-free (and normal packaged food) as much as possible

- If you want to eat corn chips, tortillas, or have corn flour, try to find a brand that is organic to start with, and labeled as non-GMO if possible

- Eat it sparingly, as if it's a treat, and not part of a regular diet

Time to Get
Label Savvy

Reading the backs of labels will be an integral part of your life now. As I mentioned earlier, I spent hours upon hours in the grocery store my first few times trying to decipher the chemical shit storm on the products' labels. The more I studied labels, the more shocked I was to find out just how much crap was put into gluten-free food. But before we delve into that, let's look at how to spot a product with gluten or gluten derivatives. This is integral not only to ensure you never consume gluten, but also makes life easier and find better alternatives.

Each country has a different law that surrounds how ingredients and additives are to be labeled on food packaging. I've listed below the codes in Australia and the US to give you a comparison and strongly recommend you research the labeling laws in your own country. This is also handy to know when traveling.

Australian labeling laws

Australia has the most stringent labeling laws in the world, which is great; however, they don't have nearly as many amazing products as the US and UK. Australian Labelling Law states:

1. Foods labeled as "gluten-free" must not contain any detectable gluten; and no oats or oat derived products; or cereals containing gluten that have used malt or malt derivatives.

2. Ingredients derived from gluten-containing grains must be declared on the food label, however small the amount.

3. Foods labeled as "low gluten" must contain less than 200 parts per million of gluten (0.02%).

4. Food labels must list all allergens. Gluten is one of them.

5. Food labels must state if the food has been processed in a facility that processes other allergen-containing foods.

As Australian labeling is so strict, sometimes it can be a little confusing for celiacs. To give you an example, consider glucose syrup.

Glucose syrup is derived from wheat. However, the Coeliac Society of Australia[67] states that it can be safe to eat. However, food labeling laws previously required the label to indicate the product contains wheat, even if it does not contain any detectable gluten and can technically be labeled gluten-free. However, now this has been reviewed and providing that the syrup contains less than 20 ppm (parts per million), the label does not need to state whether or not it's wheat derived. This one can be exceptionally confusing.

There are 10 significant allergens required to be labeled on Australian and New Zealand food products:

- Grains containing gluten, namely wheat, rye, barley, oats, and spelt

- Added sulfites in concentrations of greater than 10mg/kg

- Crustacea (shellfish)
- Milk

- Eggs
- Peanuts

- Fish
- Soybeans

- Sesame seeds
- Tree nuts

When I read food labels in Australia, I look immediately for the words *gluten* and *wheat*. It's easy, as all allergens must be listed in **bold**. After the ingredients' list, the label must also state on a separate line, "Contains...."

---

[67] www.coeliac.org.au

Below are two examples of food product labels in Australia that highlight the allergens. The first is regular wheat cookies packaged without any *free-from* labeling.

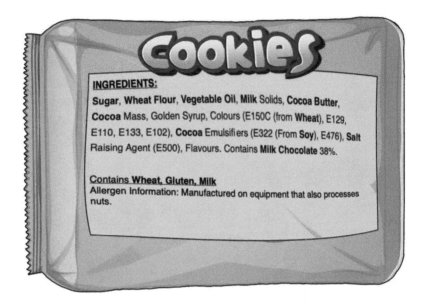

This next label is from a package of ice cream labeled gluten-free.

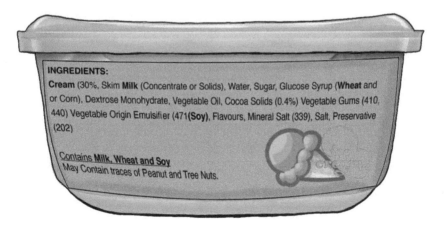

So, as you can see from the two examples, the first label clearly shows both wheat and gluten, and the second label is of a product that is technically gluten-free yet it still indicates wheat. Due to the *'overly specific'* guidelines in Australia, I've found this has made it quite confusing to people.

This product does not contain gluten; however, it contains wheat-derived products. Would I still eat this product? Nope, I won't. The reason? For a start, glucose syrup isn't good for you, along with the soy, vegetable oils, gums, mineral salts, and preservatives. Not to mention what if one day you forgot to double check a product for gluten free vs wheat free and accidentally glutened yourself? It's not worth the risk. There are better alternatives available and I show you how to find them in the chapter **How to Spot Healthy Gluten-Free Products.**

My simple rule is: if the product contains either wheat or gluten, then do not eat it. This way, you won't have to remember types of additives like glucose syrup and you won't run the risk of getting caught out.

United States labeling laws

I have to give the US credit; there are new rules surrounding the labeling of products and one of them goes beyond just identifying gluten-containing products. Manufacturers can include labeling if the product is free of genetically modified ingredients. I wish we had that in Australia. Avoiding GMO food is just one more step we can take toward healing the body as corn and soy are some of the most highly genetically modified crops in the world, and they happen to make up the bulk of gluten-free foods.

There are eight food allergens defined in the USA:

- Wheat
- Crustacean
- Eggs
- Fish
- Milk
- Peanuts
- Soybeans
- Tree nuts

Labelling a food product gluten-free is voluntary, but it comes with the stipulations listed below.

1. To label a food product gluten-free, it must:

    a. be naturally gluten-free

    b. not contain an ingredient from a gluten-containing grain

c. not contain an ingredient from a gluten-containing grain that *has not* been processed to remove the gluten (like wheat flour)

d. not contain an ingredient derived from a gluten-containing grain that *has* been processed to remove the gluten (like wheat starch) but results in the food containing more than 20ppm of gluten

2. To be labeled gluten-free the product must contain 20 parts per million (0.002%) or less of gluten.

3. Manufacturers are required to label food products that are made with an ingredient that is a major food allergen in one of the ways shown below.

Nutrition Facts

Ingredients: Enriched flour (wheat flour, malted barley, niacin, reduced iron, thiamin mononitrate, riboflavin, folic acid), sugar, partially hydrogenated cottonseed oil, high fructose corn syrup, whey (milk), eggs, vanilla, natural and artificial flavoring, salt, leavening (sodium acid pyrophosphate, monocalcium phosphate), lecithin (soy), mono- and diglycerides.

Any Cookie Company
College Park, MD 20740

1. Include the name of the food source in parenthesis following the common or usual name of the major food allergen in the list of ingredients in instances when the name of the food source of the major food allergen does not appear elsewhere in the ingredient statement for another allergenic ingredient.

2. Place the word "Contains," followed by the name of the food source from which the major food allergen is derived, immediately after or adjacent to the list of ingredients, in a type size that is no smaller than that used for the ingredient list.

Nutrition Facts

Ingredients: Enriched flour (wheat flour, malted barley, niacin, reduced iron, thiamin mononitrate, riboflavin, folic acid), sugar, partially hydrogenated cottonseed oil, high fructose corn syrup, whey, eggs, vanilla, natural and artificial flavoring, salt, leavening (sodium acid pyrophosphate, monocalcium phosphate), lecithin, mono- and diglycerides.

Contains: Wheat, Milk, Egg and Soy.

Any Cookie Company
College Park, MD 20740

Country comparison

So, you can see clear differences.

Australia allows a product to be labeled gluten-free if it does not contain gluten but does contain a wheat derived ingredient, whereas the USA does not. I have a pizza dough from Italy that is labeled gluten-free, but its main ingredient is wheat starch. This product can be labeled as gluten-free in Australia, but not the USA.

In the labeling, another difference between Australia and the USA is the fact that Australia lists gluten as a major allergen, not just wheat, and therefore, it is displayed differently. The USA allows foods with up to 0.002% gluten to be labeled as gluten-free, whereas in Australia the food cannot have any detectable gluten whatsoever.

Anything that is labeled with wheat in the USA should be avoided, whereas anything labeled with gluten should be avoided in Australia.

Chapter 13

E-Number
Nasties

G luten-free products are not always what they seem. Understanding that it *doesn't* contain gluten is one thing, but what about understanding what it *does* contain? Just because it says *gluten-free* doesn't mean it's healthy for you. Part of reading labels may require you to learn what E-Numbers are depending on which country you are in.

In Australia, labels can contain a lot of numbers starting with "E" followed by a series of digits. The "E" simply stands for *European*, as the Europeans developed a system for food additive classification. Each additive number has an "E-number" assigned.

Australia has adopted this system. You might see some labels with only an E-number, or sometimes an E-number with the full additive name after it or just the name. I find it very useful and quick to read labels in Australia as it's easier to remember E-numbers than a super long clinical name. For example, E1442 is easier to remember than hydroxypropyl distarch phosphate.

The USA has not adopted this same system and they list the full additive name, so it requires a lot more learning.

The following is a list of what I call *E-Number Nasties*. These are the top additives I avoid at all costs and you'll soon see the reasons why. You can download a comprehensive cheat sheet you can print and take a photo of. Just head to www.thegfhub.com website to download a copy.

E102 Yellow 4 - Tartrazine

Purpose: Food coloring; used to color drinks, sweets, jams, cereals, snack foods, canned fish, packaged soups, yogurt, cosmetics, wasabi, birth control pills.

Risks/Side Effects: Tartrazine is derived from coal and has been labeled literally as *industrial waste*. It has been known to provoke asthma attacks and is linked to thyroid tumors, chromosomal damage, and hives. It is banned in Norway and Austria.

E110 Yellow 3 - Sunset Yellow FCF

Purpose: Food coloring; used in cereals, bakery, sweets, snack food, ice cream, drinks, canned fish, medications, effervescent vitamins, cosmetics, hand sanitizers, mouth wash.

Risks/Side Effects: Yellow 3 is manufactured from petrochemicals (petroleum or gas) and has been known to result in hives, runny nose, allergies, kidney tumors, hyperactivity, abdominal pain, vomiting, indigestion, and swollen eyelids. It is banned in Norway.

E120 - Carmine

Purpose: Coloring; used in dairy, sweets, drinks, ice creams, cosmetics.

Risks/Side Effects: Produced from some insects or the aluminum salt of some acids, it can cause adverse reactions in asthmatics, and produces rashes, vomiting, and triggers an allergic response. It is banned in Belgium, Switzerland, Sweden, Austria, and Norway.

E221 - Sodium Sulfite

Purpose: Preservative; used in wine and dried fruit.

Risks/Side Effects: Sodium sulfite is a soluble salt that is a byproduct of sulfur dioxide. It can cause issues for asthmatics and induce headaches, breathing problems, wheezing, and rashes.

My personal note: I love wine. I don't want to give it up because of sulfites, yet I do feel the effects of sulfites the next day. I get bad headaches and a very dry mouth. Interestingly enough, this happens mostly with Australian and New Zealand wines, not so much with European wines, even though they still contain sulfites. The unfortunate thing about sulfite labeling is that you don't know what quantity is used. So, when possible I try to find an organic sulfite-free wine. There is a little trick I use and it's called *hydrogen peroxide*. Most people might think of hydrogen peroxide as a bleach for hair or even as nasty cleaning chemical, and while it can be used for those things, it's simply H20 (water) with an added hydrogen molecule. This has strong oxidative properties and it's also a component of living cells. When used in large concentrations, you can certainly bleach with it, but when used in the right quantities, it can neutralize sulfites in wine. I have two little bottles of it that I purchased from a liquor store, one for at home, and the other for my handbag when dining out. I add five drops into a whole bottle of wine or one drop per glass. That's enough to do the trick for me. I'm not trying to sell it to you, but if you want to read more about it, here's the link to the product I use: https://www.purewine.com.au. I have no affiliation with this company, by the way. I think it's very tactful for a winemaker to invent a product like this so people like me keep drinking wine, so hey, I'm not complaining.

E250 - Sodium Nitrate

Purpose: Preservative; used in cured meats and fish products.

Risks/Side Effects: Sodium nitrate is an alkali metal nitrate salt that is used to manufacture fertilizer, fireworks, smoke bombs, glass, and pottery enamels. It's also used to keep your cured meats fresh. It's been linked to Alzheimer's, diabetes, Parkinson's, and various types of cancer.

E320/E321 - BHA & BHT (Butylated hydroxyanisole & butylated hydroxytoluene)

Purpose: Synthetic antioxidant; protects fat-related products like chewing gum, margarine, and potato chips against rancidity.

Risks/Side Effects: A petroleum derivative that has known to cause hyperactivity, is a known carcinogen, creates estrogenic effects, and vitamin and mineral imbalances. It is banned in Japan, the UK, and most European countries.

E464 - Hydroxypropyl Methyl Cellulose

Purpose: Emulsifier and gum. It is a chemically modified wood cellulose that is used in tile adhesives, cement renders, paint, cosmetics, and detergents. It is used to thicken foods like GF bread and gravies.

Risks/Side Effects: When consumed in large quantities, it ferments in the large intestine and can cause intestinal problems such as bloating, constipation, and diarrhea.

E512 - Stannous Chloride

Purpose: Antioxidant. Stannous Chloride is a white crystalline solid prepared from tin ores and hydrochloric acid. It is used as a thickening agent in canned beans and asparagus.

Risks/Side Effects: Known to cause nausea, headaches, and gastric upsets.

E621 - Monosodium Glutamate[68]

Purpose: Flavor enhancer; used to enhance flavor in canned foods, meat, dry products, powders, gravies, seasonings. Has a salty taste. You will probably remember the whole *Chinese food MSG saga*. I do, and I remember not being allowed to go to my favorite Chinese restaurant because my mother said, "*They put MSG in the food to make you full.*" She was partially correct, but everyone seemed to forget that. Rather, food companies began labeling products with MSG, and they tricked customers by only listing the E-number or the technical term *Monosodium Glutamate* so most people wouldn't realize what they were eating.

Risks/Side Effects: There are more and more people reporting issues with MSG, including migraines, chest pain, weight gain, brain damage, and liver inflammation. I personally know a celiac friend who is an MSG detector. If she eats anything with MSG, she suffers immense migraines very quickly that last a long time. The poor thing suffers! It's still used in many restaurants in their gravies and spice blends today.

E927a - Azodicarbonamide

Purpose: Improving agent; commonly used in plastics, yoga mats, shoe soles, etc. It is also used as a flour bleacher and dough conditioner.

Risks/Side Effects: It is linked to asthma and can exacerbate allergy symptoms. It is banned in the UK, Europe, and Australia but is still used commonly

---

[68] Niaz, K., Zaplatic, E., and Spoor, J. (2018). "Extensive use of monosodium glutamate: A threat to public health?". EXCLI J, 17:273-278. doi:10.17179/excli2018-1092

in foods in the US like English muffins. They can be found in Wendy's™ sandwiches, Arby's™ burgers, and even Starbucks™ croissants.

E951 - Aspartame

Purpose: Artificial sweetener; commonly used in Coke™, cereals, chewing gums, mints, toothpaste, deserts. It's sold under the name NutraSweet™ and Equal™ for retail purchase. Many companies will claim that a product is *sugar-free* but put this bad boy in instead.

Risks/Side Effects: Aspartame is a neurotoxin (toxic to the brain tissues) and is carcinogenic (cancer causing.) It is known to affect short term memory and erode intelligence and may lead to ailments such as Parkinson's, multiple sclerosis, brain tumors, lymphoma, diabetes, chronic fatigue, depression, anxiety attacks, dizziness, headaches, and nausea.

E1442 -Hydroxypropyl Distarch Phosphate

Purpose: Modified starch / thickener; commonly the first and main ingredient in gluten-free alternative food. Used as a gluten-free alternative flour.

Risks/side Effects: Digestive system.

Typically, this starch is produced from genetically modified corn or potato starch but it is also from tapioca starch. The starch's structure and properties are changed by dissolving it in water, exposing it to a variety of acids, and going through an evaporation process that turns the liquid to a fine white powder that smells like vinegar. It is now resistant to high temperatures and frost. When the finished powder is dissolved in water for use in food products, its volume increases largely.

The tapioca starch version is created with propylene oxide, which is used to make plastic and is a probable human carcinogen, and phosphoric acid which is used for a wide variety of things like a rust inhibitor, fertilizer, feedstock, and home cleaning products.

These modified starches are widely used in creams, snacks, freezer meals, long life shelf items, soups, sausages, flours, cookie mixes etc. You would be surprised to know that it also lurks in baby food!

There is no regulation on the safe production of this additive and there is no regulation as to the concentration it's allowed to be used in. Studies of the effects of this modified starch are continuing. So far, the side effects reported include nausea, vomiting, bloating, slow digestion of food, gastrointestinal tract disturbance, inflammation, aggravation of ulcers, and gastritis.

Please go to my website www.thegfhub.com for a free downloadable *E-Nasties Cheat Sheet* that explains more numbers to watch out for. Also, refer to the resource section at the back of this book. But if you're like me and sometimes struggle to remember all this information, I've made a miniature version of the cheat sheet to take with you in your handbag/man-bag. When you come to reading labels on food products, you can quickly and easily whip out your cheat sheet and see if any of the numbers on the package match your sheet, and if they do, then I would suggest putting that product back and finding a healthier alternative.

How Starches and Additives
in GF Foods Affect the Body

ow, so far there has been a lot to take in with learning how to detect gluten, learning about sugar, soy & corn, reading labels, and a crash course on nasty food additives. Let's put this all together and break down common gluten-free products and learn how the starches and additives can affect the body.

The first issue with having to remove gluten/wheat from your diet is finding suitable replacements. Gluten has a remarkable structure: it's so elastic, rather indestructible, expands easily, and holds its form. It's so unique that no other grain can compete with this combination of properties.

When yeast is added to a typical gluten-based bread, it makes the dough rise by producing gas bubbles during baking. Gluten is strong enough that it expands around these bubbles and prevents the bread from falling or sagging. Most flours used to make bread are made of refined four, where the bran (outer layer) and germ (seed for the new plant) are removed and all that's left is the starchy part of the grain. This results in a light and airy texture.

To achieve something similar to the flexibility and lightness of wheat bread, we need to find an ingredient to bind the fibers together so they don't fall apart and use starches to achieve the lightness. If you did a straight one-for-one replacement of wheat flour with sorghum flour, and baked muffins using the same recipe, you would find that the sorghum muffins would be heavy like soccer balls or just crumble after baking. The reason is that there is no glue holding it together and no elasticity to make it light and springy. The whole grain is much heavier than the refined starch from wheat.

In gluten-free alternative food, the main substitutes are soy, rice, corn, tapioca, and modified starches. Most companies' recipes will use a combination of refined and modified starches to achieve the light and fluffy aspect, and gums to bind the fibers together.

However, excess starches are very unhealthy, and gums can cause stomach upsets. Let's look at starch and why it's important to understand the differences between starches and flours.

Starch in a whole food, like a baked potato, is an excellent source of carbohydrates and is nutritious in vitamins and minerals, provided you don't add tons of bacon bits and sour cream. The potato *is* a high carbohydrate food but eaten as a whole includes the right balance of fiber to aid in digestion. I personally love potatoes; they're one of my favorite vegetables. I'm practically a potato addict.

Now take that potato, remove the fiber, extract the starch content and you will have a light powdery mixture to work with. However, cooking with this starch means there is no fiber in your muffins. So, using it as the main ingredient in your muffin or bread mix, combined with other refined starches like tapioca and corn starch...what does it now give you? A nutrient-void product that can cause inflammation, convert very quickly to sugars in your body, and deposit fat right on your ass. It will trigger your poor pancreas to work harder to release insulin into your blood to deal with this highly refined, starchy product.

Touching back to what we learned in Anatomy 101 and earlier in the book, your pancreas measures the amount of sugar in your blood. When it senses the sugar levels are too high, it releases insulin into the blood, which then stores those carbohydrates in your cells to be used later. Problem is, most of us don't use the stored energy later. It turns to fat and we just keep getting fatter and fatter. The insulin level in your blood should look like the rolling waves of the ocean, but when you eat high-carbohydrate foods, like bread for breakfast, sandwiches and bagels for lunch, then pasta for dinner, your insulin level looks like constant peaks and valleys. Your body doesn't get a chance to rest and if this keeps up, you can develop insulin resistance.

Starches, especially modified starches, are just as dangerous as injecting pure sugar into your blood. Starches are supposed to be consumed with fiber and not in its pure straight form.

To put this in perspective for you, here is an equation to help you understand how starch equates to sugar in the body.

(Total Carbs minus the fiber) ÷ by 5 = the teaspoon equivalent of sugar

Let's look at flour

Let's look at a label of an off-the-shelf gluten-free flour product.

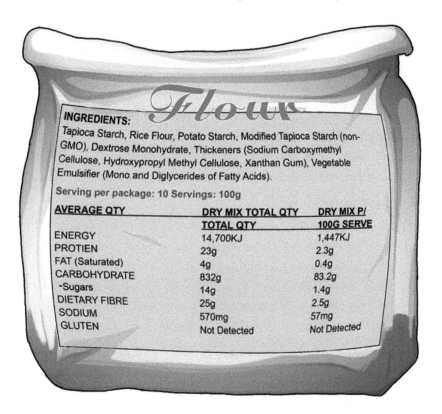

You can probably already identify the issues with this product, but let's break it down.

The order of the ingredients listed on labels are from the highest concentration to the least concentration.

Tapioca Starch—Refined starch causes inflammation and converts to sugars quickly in the body.

Rice Flour—It doesn't state here whether it is white rice or brown rice. At a guess, I would say white rice flour, as the flour color is pure white. White rice is highly refined and nowhere near as good or healthy as its counterpart brown rice.

Potato Starch—again refined starch causes inflammation and converts to sugars quickly in the body.

Modified Tapioca Starch (E1442)—The mega-nasty chemical monster that you've learned about in the E-numbers.

Dextrose Monohydrate—A simple sugar produced by the hydrolysis of starch. Typically, dextrose monohydrate is derived from corn. However, the description on this product's website says there is 'no added corn' so it's unknown what the source is. Regardless, it's a highly refined, highly processed simple sugar.

Thickeners: Sodium Carboxymethyl Cellulose (E466) / Hydroxypropyl Methyl Cellulose (E464)—These are prepared from wood cellulose and plant structures. It's used as a filler and an anti-clumping agent. It is plant-based; however, it can ferment in the large intestine and large concentrations can cause bloating, constipation, and diarrhea.

Xanthan Gum (E415)—A natural, plant-based gum derived from the fermentation of corn sugar with a bacterium. This is used to help bind substances together. People have reported feelings of bloating, constipation, and diarrhea just as with the other two thickeners. You will see the use of gums in a lot of store-bought gluten-free flours and recipes as they are needed to help glue the flour together in baking. There are alternatives like flaxseed, eggs, and psyllium husk.

Emulsifier: Mono- and Diglyceride fatty acids—These can be animal- or plant-based. It is used as an emulsifier and there are no known adverse side effects. However, it's another additive. You will also notice there is very little protein and the little bit there would have come from the rice flour.

As you can see, this product is predominately made of *starch* rather than whole grain milled flour. The impact on your body is significant, so much so that 100g of this product is equal to 16 teaspoons of sugar!!!

Total carbohydrates of this flour: 83.2g per 100g.

Fiber: 2.5g.

$(83.2 - 2.5) \div 5 = 16.14$ teaspoons of sugar per 100g

For the entire 1kg (2.2lb) bag, you have 161.4 teaspoons of sugar effect. One teaspoon of sugar is equal to about 5g of carbs and 20 calories. A 1kg bag of flour has over 3,220 calories in it.

That's equivalent to 10.7 McDonald's cheeseburgers!

Here is a label from a traditional bag of organic spelt wheat flour.

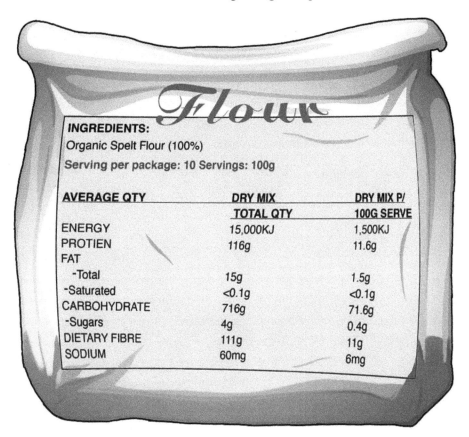

INGREDIENTS:
Organic Spelt Flour (100%)
Serving per package: 10 Servings: 100g

AVERAGE QTY	DRY MIX TOTAL QTY	DRY MIX P/ 100G SERVE
ENERGY	15,000KJ	1,500KJ
PROTIEN	116g	11.6g
FAT		
-Total	15g	1.5g
-Saturated	<0.1g	<0.1g
CARBOHYDRATE	716g	71.6g
-Sugars	4g	0.4g
DIETARY FIBRE	111g	11g
SODIUM	60mg	6mg

For a start, there is only one ingredient (not nine like the gluten-free flour). We can see that the protein content is far greater due to the gluten, yet the carbohydrates and sugars are *less*. There are no other additives, gums, emulsifiers, thickeners, or chemical sugars added. Per 100g of flour there is the equivalent of 12 teaspoons of sugar, compared to the 16 teaspoons of the gluten-free flour.

It's a double-edged sword. Gluten causes havoc to the body, even in individuals who are not celiac or gluten intolerant. However, swapping to a generic commercial brand gluten-free flour can be just as bad. When looking for a suitable flour alternative, we really want to find a product composed of flour *more* than starch.

Flour is just the vegetable (like potato or buckwheat groats) dried and ground up as a whole. It retains its fiber, protein, and starch, and is much more digestible to the body and more nutritious.

Starch is a flavorless white powder used as a thickening agent. It comes from a multi-step process of extracting the starch from the vegetable. Yes, it creates lightness to your baked goods, but it's nutrient-void and converts quickly to sugars in the body. Modified starch is the worst of the worst.

You may find that, to achieve a desirable outcome, you might not be able to substitute wheat flour for just one kind of alternative flour (like buckwheat.) You may need a blend of different flours that you can buy or make yourself.

Sometimes you might just have to use a starch to create that perfect fluffy blueberry and white chocolate muffin. If that's the case, use plain starch (not modified) and in small quantities. Ensure that the flour content outweighs the starch content. Incorporating more whole grain flours into your recipes will help to maintain fullness and assist with your digestion.

Not to dampen the mood, but gluten-free flour is not as easy as you think. There are so many recipes that call for gluten-free flour and magically, the picture of the food looks sumptuous. But hang on, there are 50 million varieties of gluten-free flour to use. *(Ok, not 50 million, but a lot.)*

Those flours, gums, and starches all react differently. Don't get too disappointed when those fluffy blueberry and white chocolate muffins in the picture turn out like rock hard little soccer balls. It can take some practice to get the right blend.

Let's look at bread

Usually, the first thing people look for when going gluten-free is an alternative bread option. At this point, you will realize that anything with a shelf life is usually not going to be that healthy because there are so many stabilizers, fillers, and additives in it.

Essentially, store-bought bread is just the crappy commercial flour you've read about above turned into bread. It will be light and fluffy, it will look and taste similar to traditional wheat bread, but it *is* unhealthy for you.

This is an off-the-shelf loaf of gluten-free bread from a local supermarket nearby.

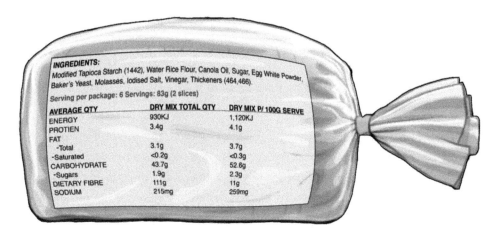

INGREDIENTS:
Modified Tapioca Starch (1442), Water Rice Flour, Canola Oil, Sugar, Egg White Powder, Baker's Yeast, Molasses, Iodised Salt, Vinegar, Thickeners (464,466).

Serving per package: 6 Servings: 83g (2 slices)

AVERAGE QTY	DRY MIX TOTAL QTY	DRY MIX P/ 100G SERVE
ENERGY	930KJ	1,120KJ
PROTIEN	3.4g	4.1g
FAT		
-Total	3.1g	3.7g
-Saturated	<0.2g	<0.3g
CARBOHYDRATE	43.7g	52.6g
-Sugars	1.9g	2.3g
DIETARY FIBRE	111g	11g
SODIUM	215mg	259mg

As you can see, the first and most highly concentrated ingredient is modified tapioca starch. That nasty horrible additive. Again, the rice flour is not identified as brown or white but is assumed white as it's white bread. Canola oil is a refined vegetable oil that causes free-radical damage. Egg white powder is used to bind; not so bad, but what's wrong with using fresh eggs? Bakers' yeast is used to make it rise. Molasses for the sweetness. Salt and vinegar are self-explanatory. Sodium carboxymethyl cellulose (E466) / hydroxypropyl methyl cellulose (E464) are thickeners.

This is an Australian product, so you can see that sometimes the full technical name of the ingredient is listed (modified tapioca starch 1442). Sometimes it's not, as the thickeners have only their E-number listed and not the additive itself. This can make things quite confusing when people want to understand what's really in their product. In the US, as mentioned, E-numbers are not widely used and the entire technical name is given instead.

There is the equivalent of 8.6 teaspoons of sugar in two slices of this bread.

This bread is light and fluffy and would work toasted or in a fresh sandwich. It looks and feels like traditional sandwich bread, but it's made of modified starches and additives. I don't consider this to be a healthy alternative.

The big giants are cashing in

The gluten-free product market size, globally, is projected to reach $13 billion USD by 2025.[69]

With more people being diagnosed with celiac disease, IBS, and gluten intolerance, the Big Giants are cashing in more than ever before. But is it at the expense of the people's health?

North America is the leading consumer market for gluten-free products, holding over a 50% share. Australia is among the most lucrative markets in the Asia Pacific, with the government issuing a helping hand to start-ups in the food and beverage industry. Bakery and dairy/meat alternatives are among the most highly produced products forecasted for growth till 2025 and the mass chains of grocery stores and merchandisers take the lead in expanding their product lines.

What does this all mean exactly?

It means that there will be an abundance of new products on the market in a short amount of time and you need to be savvy about what's healthy and what's not.

From a company perspective, they want to deliver a product that costs less to manufacture and yields more profit. It's just the nature of the beast. So, do you think big companies really care about the health and well-being of you and your family? Do you think they are inclined to use a cheap modified starch, or an organic wholegrain flour that costs more but is healthier for you? The choice will drive their profits up or down.

There are some brands of bread and flour that make traditional wheat products and are now making gluten-free alternatives. I've certainly seen countless companies manufacturing both wheat and gluten-free bread. It's a growing industry with a growing consumer market that companies want in on.

---

[69] https://www.globenewswire.com/news-release/2019/05/22/1840582

I'm not slandering companies, their ethics, or their production methods. My point to all of this is be mindful of what you put in your mouth, continue to learn about what's good for you so you can steer clear of marketing hype, unhealthy products, and mass-produced food with little nutrition.

Chapter 15

How to Spot
Healthy Gluten-Free Products

When speaking to people about the food I eat or how I make my bread, I get a lot of comments like, *"I've never heard of that flour before"* or *"I've never heard of that product before."* I know I didn't cook with sorghum, teff, and amaranth before I was diagnosed, so it was a learning process for me, too.

The flours mentioned in this section are a mixture of seeds, fruits, nuts, and grains and I explain the benefits of them all.

But let's have a little chat about grains. There is much controversy surrounding grains. The reality is, it's hard enough to avoid gluten, soy, HFCS, and nasty additives, let alone other grains. I'm sure you've heard of the grain-free movement at one time or another? Dr. Perlmutter advocates against grains and I even feed my dog grain-free food. But sometimes avoiding grains is exceptionally hard to do. So, the more you know about grains and the best method of preparing them, the better off you are if you want to eat them. Don't forget *balance* and *moderation*. What works for one, might not work for another.

I always say to people who are adopting a gluten-free lifestyle, listen to your body when you eat other grains. It will let you know how it feels.

Understand though that other grain proteins will not affect you like gluten. I've had many people tell me they respond to rice and corn the same way they do to gluten and that they are having a gluten reaction. However, protein in rice and corn does not initiate your immune response like wheat gluten and your villi are not being destroyed like they would from a gluten response. It may be the lectins in those grains that are causing the upsets, a soy allergy, and just plain inflammation, *but it's important to remember that only gluten from wheat, barley, and rye can cause degradation of the villi from an auto-immune response.*

What do good quality ingredients look like?

To find a healthy gluten-free product, you need to learn what healthy ingredients look like. Thanks to earlier chapters, you now know how to spot the nasty additives and starches, but what makes one gluten-free product a better choice over another?

Healthy Wheat Flour Alternatives		
Almond Meal	Cassava	Oat
Amaranth	Coconut	Quinoa
Besan / Chickpea	Green Banana	Sorghum
Brown Rice Flour	Masa Harina	Teff
Buckwheat	Millet	Tigernut

First, let's look at some options for healthy flour alternatives.

Coconut - fruit, nut, seed

Coconut flour is made from fresh coconut flesh. The flesh is dried, defatted, and ground into a powder that resembles flour. It is low carb, as compared to other flours, and has a high concentration of protein. It is rich in fiber and has a minimal effect on blood sugar levels.

Almond - nut

Almond flour is super simple; it's just ground almonds. Almond flour is typically made from blanched almonds (with the husk removed) and is ground more finely to a flour consistency. Almond meal, however,, is ground almonds, husk and all. Almonds contain healthy fats, minerals, and protein.

Sorghum - grain

Sorghum flour is made up of an ancient grain and is non-GMO. It's high in fiber, has a neutral flavor, and is a concentrated source of phenolic compounds (antioxidant, antiviral, and anti-inflammatory). It is great in baking and is closer to mimicking gluten compounds.

Buckwheat - seed

Buckwheat is actually a seed and is not related to wheat despite its name. The flour is made from ground up buckwheat groats which can be used as a porridge, and the flour can be used in baking and pastas. Buckwheat contains proteins, minerals, and carbs. The carbs have a minimal effect on blood sugar compared to other starches. It's also concentrated in antioxidants.

Quinoa - seed

Quinoa is a seed in the same family as buckwheat. It's harvested from a tall leafy plant that is not a grain-grass. Quinoa is crunchy and nutty and another good source of antioxidants and minerals. You can find quinoa porridge, which is the seeds rolled out or seeds popped like popcorn. Quinoa flour is simply milled up quinoa seeds, fiber and all. Quinoa comes in multiple colors with white, red, and black. (It's pronounced keen-wah not quin-oA. We don't want to look silly when asking for this at the store.)

Oat - grain

Oats are among one of the healthiest of grains, full of protein and minerals. It helps to lower cholesterol, decrease blood pressure and keeps you feeling fuller for longer.

Before you start panicking about oats, there are two sides to the story. Oats do **not** contain the same gluten protein as found in wheat. It contains a protein called *avenin sativa* or just *avenin* for short. The Coeliac Society of Australia advises to avoid oats as some celiacs may have a reaction to this protein, *but* most will not. It's reported that a very minute percentage of celiacs (less than 10%) will react to the avenin protein in oats, so it's to be used with caution after you have been gluten-free for some time. Self-testing and evaluation are required to see if you tolerate this grain. An issue with oats is cross contamination from other grains (discussed in the chapter **To oat or not to oat)**. Oat is still a grain, and there are more discussions surrounding the negative effects grains on the body in general, so it's up to you if you would like to eat a grain-free diet, or relish in the fact that you have a 90% possibility that you can still enjoy your porridge for breakfast on a cold winter's morning.

Besan/Chickpea - legume

Besan flour, also known as gram or garbanzo, is made from ground up dried chickpeas. It is commonly used in Indian cuisine and is super rich in folate, copper, and manganese. It's full of vitamins and minerals, has fewer calories than regular flour, keeps you feeling fuller for longer, and has a minimal effect on blood sugar levels. It has a mild nutty flavor that works well in most baked goods.

Cassava - vegetable

Cassava is a root vegetable or tuber with a nutty flavor. Originating in South America, it's a major product consumed in developing countries. Cassava in the US is also referred to as yuca or Brazilian arrowroot. Cassava is high in carbs and low in fiber, vitamins, and minerals compared to the other flours and should be used sparingly. Cassava flour is made up from the root. If you have heard of tapioca, that is the starch made from refining the starch content from the cassava root.

Teff - grain

Teff is an ancient grain with a nutty almost hazelnut flavor and a moist texture. Traditionally teff has been used to make a fermented sourdough flatbread   called injera in Africa. The teff grain is ground up into flour and comes in two colors, brown and ivory. Teff is a cut above quinoa, having more calcium, fiber, zinc, and thiamine. The teff grain can be used in porridge and stews.

Masa Harina - grain

Masa harina translated from Spanish means *dough flour*. It's made from corn that is dried then treated in a solution of lime and water. The lime reacts with the niacin in the corn to make it more digestible. The soaked corn is then washed and ground into masa and once dried it's called masa harina. When you add water, it returns to its dough-like consistency. Masa harina is used in a lot of Mexican dishes for tortillas, tamales, and empanadas. It's an excellent source of fiber and contains beneficial vitamins and minerals.

Brown Rice - grain

This is mostly self-explanatory. Milled up brown rice equals brown rice flour. It is a fantastic substitute for wheat flour and a great source of fiber, but it is lower in folate and has fewer phytonutrients than wheat flour.

Make sure you buy your brown rice flour from a reputable source. I was caught out at the store buying a product labeled *brown rice flour* but the ingredients were actually white rice (88%) with added bran (12%). Rice is one grain; it starts off as brown rice but is turned into white rice when the bran and germ are removed. The bran and germ contain essential vitamins and minerals so if you end up buying a product that is white rice with bran added, you're missing out on the whole grain. Best to make sure you're getting what you pay for and what you want is whole ground brown rice.

Millet - grain

This is one of the lesser known grains in western cultures, although it's been around in Asia and India for nearly 10,000 years. It comes in a variety of colors (white, yellow, grey, and red) and in different grain sizes. You can roast it, cook it like rice, and even mash it like potatoes. It is loaded with folate, choline, magnesium, phosphorus, and zinc. It has an amazing ability to reduce starch absorption, so it carries a minimal effect on blood sugar levels.

Amaranth - seed

Amaranth has been around for over 8,000 years and was considered a staple in Aztec civilizations. Amaranth is packed with manganese, magnesium, phosphorus, and iron. Studies have shown that amaranth could have an anti-inflammatory effect on the body. You can add the grains to smoothies, use it instead of rice or couscous, mix it into stews to add thickness, or mill the groats up into flour for baking.

Green Banana - fruit

Green banana flour again is another uncommon ingredient in most households. However, for the people of the Caribbean and Africa it's a well-known staple. Green banana flour is exactly that, dried up green (unripened) bananas milled into flour. Even though ripe bananas have a very distinct taste, green banana flour when cooked is rather earthy, neutral, and mild in comparison. It's great for sweet and savory dishes. Green banana flour is a resistant starch which is a fermentable fiber that passes through the intestines undigested and is a fantastic source of probiotics. It's high in minerals and 5HTP (5-hydroxytryptophan) which helps to increase serotonin production, so you can get a dose of natural antidepressant effects from this flour.

Finding the best alternatives

So, now you can see all the beneficial vitamins, minerals, nutrients, and fiber in these alternatives. Why would you want to choose something that's made up of pure starch?

Good alternatives aren't always going to be in your local grocery store. I know mine only stock a basic like brown rice four, and if I want anything else listed here, I have to buy it from a health food store or order it online. Some larger chain stores might have a *health food* aisle and yes, they will contain many gluten-free options. But are they good quality or not?

My local grocery store chain, Coles™, has its very own line of GF alternative food called *Free-From*. However, the majority of it is mass-produced, full of starch, additives, and soybean oils that I don't consider to be healthy. I have found major chain supermarkets don't tend to stock smaller boutique products as these smaller suppliers may not be able to keep up with the demand to fill all the chain stores in the nation. Usually, the healthier it is, the shorter the shelf life. Therefore, rolling out these products across a nationwide chain may not be a profitable option for them.

Start by finding out what your local grocery store does carry. Then get out of your comfort zone, put your hippy pants on, and make friends with your health food shop! See what options they offer. If you need to grab items from the health food store and it's not close by, purchase in bulk. Don't buy one packet, buy three! There's nothing worse than having to run to four different stores last minute before entertaining guests that night.

If you're in Australia, go to Mrs. Flannery's™ or a Go-Vita™ store.

If you're in the US, go to Whole Foods™ and Trader Joe's™. Whole Foods™, now owned by Amazon™, offers online shopping with a 2-day delivery inside the US. How easy is that?

If you're in the UK, get friendly with Planet Organic, and if you don't have one close, they have a fantastic online store as well.

If you're anywhere else in the world, I recommend iHerb.com. It's a great online retailer that ships to 150 countries worldwide. Their products can be filtered by gluten free, cruelty free, diary free, and heaps more. I use this retailer quite a lot to find amazing bath and body products that the shelves of Australian shops just don't stock. Usually shipping takes 10 days, but I'm ok to wait.

> Head to **www.iherb.com** and if you use this code **AOS6454** when you check out, you will receive an instant 5% off your purchase for as many purchases as you like and 10% of any of the iherb exclusive products.

I've spent a lot of time in the US and, like a teenage girl is to One-Direction, I'm a massive fan of Whole Foods™. I'd live in Whole Foods™ if I could and practically do whenever I'm there as it's my local go-to for lunch and dinner.

Some companies like Whole Foods™ have strict requirements about what products are even allowed to be sold in their stores, which I think is amazing. I love their philosophy and the care behind their rules and regulations, which makes shopping there a whole lot easier than shopping at Albertson's™ or Woolworths™.

My point about pulling out the old hippy pants — those stores (Wholefoods™, Mrs. Flannery's™ & Planet Organics™) have trained, helpful staff who really care about your well-being and understand food allergies. They only stock premium products that meet a specific protocol and culture. They have standards and when I've met owners of the stores, they typically have had a health or food issue themselves that led them to create the store in the first place. Some of those stores have naturopaths working there, and some even have special allergy testing, blood analysis, and many weird and wonderful hippy-healthy things to help you on your journey.

Once you have gone through the process of discovering what products you can get, like and what you want to use in your regular routine, life will become much easier. At first I kept a list in my phone of my favorite products from different stores, and now that I've shopped them so much, I know exactly which aisle and shelf they are on, so doing the regular shopping routine *of grab this and that* is rather effortless. It's become a new mind-set and one more step in an easier direction to managing this gluten-free life.

It costs *how* much to eat gluten-free?

The shocking reality of gluten-free food is it's expensive as hell! For me to buy 500 grams (roughly 1lb) of gluten-free blended alternative flour costs

$11.95AUD[70] on average. Whereas I can get the same amount of wheat flour for $0.75AUD.

Here are a few other examples:

- Simple brown rice flour is $5.95AUD.

- A loaf of artisan fresh wheat sourdough costs $7.50AUD while a nice loaf of gluten-free bread can cost up to $13.50AUD.

- Garlic bread was $1.49AUD and now its gluten-free counterpart is $3.99AUD.

Some products even carry what I call the *GF tax,* meaning they are crappy products with a high price tag simply because it says gluten-free. Many good gluten-free foods or alternative grains are more expensive because they are not mass-produced. Therefore, production costs are higher. They need to be contaminant-free in processing, which also carries a higher production cost as factories are processing less than their regular grain style counterparts.

Would you believe that celiacs in Ireland get a tax deduction/relief on gluten-free food? Italy gives out vouchers to up for 140 Euros per month to help with the cost of GF food! Australians and Americans get...*nothing*!

When first shopping for gluten-free food, you will really notice the difference in your wallet. But soon you will make adjustments, find the right products that work for you, buy when items are on sale, buy in bulk, and make a lot of your own food at home. It will just take time.

What do good quality products look like?

In the previous chapter, you saw what a crappy loaf of gluten-free bread looks like. It's full of modified starch, vegetable oil, and thickeners, and has the equivalent to 4 teaspoons of sugar per slice.

So, what does a good quality loaf of gluten-free bread look like in comparison?

Here is a copy of the label from one of my favorite breads. It's made by a small company and is sold in health food stores.

---

[70] In October 2019, $1AUD = $0.68USD.

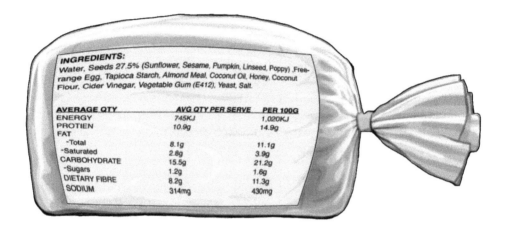

INGREDIENTS:
Water, Seeds 27.5% (Sunflower, Sesame, Pumpkin, Linseed, Poppy) ,Free-range Egg, Tapioca Starch, Almond Meal, Coconut Oil, Honey, Coconut Flour, Cider Vinegar, Vegetable Gum (E412), Yeast, Salt.

AVERAGE QTY	AVG QTY PER SERVE	PER 100G
ENERGY	745KJ	1,020KJ
PROTIEN	10.9g	14.9g
FAT		
-Total	8.1g	11.1g
-Saturated	2.8g	3.9g
CARBOHYDRATE	15.5g	21.2g
-Sugars	1.2g	1.6g
DIETARY FIBRE	8.2g	11.3g
SODIUM	314mg	430mg

The first thing you will notice is that seeds make up the most highly concentrated part of the ingredients. Free range egg is excellent; it's not a cheap caged or powdered egg. Tapioca starch is NOT modified tapioca starch; this is just plain starch. It is also not the main ingredient and is halfway down the list, so it's in a smaller concentration compared to other breads. Almond meal—*Woohoo!*—means lots of protein. Coconut oil is a wonderful source of fatty acids. Coconut flour is a great source of fiber. Cider vinegar is great for the gut and guar gum, used as a binder and in small quantities, is fine.

All the ingredients are clean, wonderfully healthy ingredients and I just love this product. Compared to the other gluten-free loaf full of starch, this bread only equates to 0.73 teaspoons of sugar equivalent, not 4. It is a denser bread, but that's the trade off if you want something healthy.

Here's the kicker: when I buy this bread, it's sold in the freezer at the health food store as it basically doesn't have a shelf life (well 2 to 3 days, they say.) The reason for this is that it contains no preservatives. It's just plain, wholesome food. This is what I deem as a great GF alternative. My only issue is…the cost! It's $13.50AUD. Now, I know that looks expensive and it is compared to the other gluten-free bread from the chain supermarket, which costs roughly $6.95. But when you break it down, it's about $1.00 per slice. If I have two slices for breakfast with some avocado on top that's a very cheap breakfast, coming in at $3.50. If you're comparing this cost with what a bowl of fruit loops costs, then throw this book out and give up now!

So, that's got bread covered. What about a flour alternative? You can buy good quality flour blends that contain grains, like sorghum and teff, and you can buy grain-free flour blends as well. Here is an example of a great quality gluten-free flour, and it happens to be grain-free.

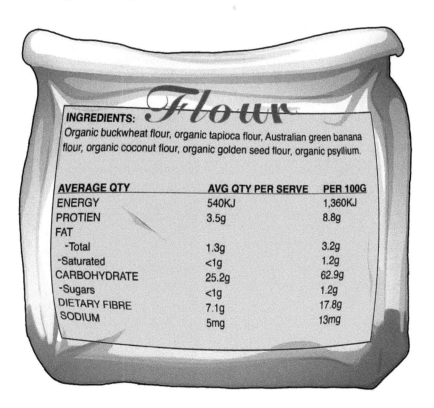

INGREDIENTS:
Organic buckwheat flour, organic tapioca flour, Australian green banana flour, organic coconut flour, organic golden seed flour, organic psyllium.

AVERAGE QTY	AVG QTY PER SERVE	PER 100G
ENERGY	540KJ	1,360KJ
PROTIEN	3.5g	8.8g
FAT		
-Total	1.3g	3.2g
-Saturated	<1g	1.2g
CARBOHYDRATE	25.2g	62.9g
-Sugars	<1g	1.2g
DIETARY FIBRE	7.1g	17.8g
SODIUM	5mg	13mg

This product is from a woman by the name of Monica Topliss, an Australia chef and proud celiac. *(I needed to mock up the label so I don't get in trouble for copyright)*.

When I was first looking for a gluten-free flour alternative, I came across this product. As I read the labels of her products, it surprised me to see that she didn't once use any starches or additives. She offers a range of flour blends for different purposes, along with a heap of other gluten-free food options. The downside is that this flour blend costs $13.50 per 400g packet. Ouch!

But as the age old saying goes, you get what you pay for.

On another packet of her flour blend an ingredient of *baking powder* was listed. Being celiac, you really need to be wary about which baking powders you use. I was sure it was fine, but I contacted her and asked her if she could break it down for me, so I understood what was in the baking powder. Within a couple of days, she emailed me back a full specification sheet from the manufacturer. Not sure why I doubted it, but what made me feel all warm and fuzzy was that this very busy chef and producer of food took the time to respond to my little request. Visit www.glutenfreefoodco.com to see more of her products.

This is an example of a small boutique company in my local town that produces fantastic quality products from a person suffering with celiac disease. You might not find this kind of boutique, quality product in the major chain stores, so get down to your local health food store to see what it has to offer.

If you are already experienced at a gluten-free lifestyle, do you have any products you could recommend? If so, please email the details to me or post it on our Facebook group.

> *Note: This is not a paid advertisement, nor am I sponsored to write about this product. None of these companies will know I have written about them until I send them a copy of this book and say, "Hey, guess what? You made it into my book. Wanna buy a copy?" Plus, most of you are overseas and can't get some products I'm mentioning. I'm just simply sharing with you some great products I've come across, and what they are made of, so you know how to find something just as good.*

What about some other staples?

Pasta, that wonderful variety of rubbery goodness in Italian food. Finding a great pasta choice can be a bit difficult, depending on your dietary issues and whether you're grain-free. Most pastas on the market are made up of grains like corn and rice. Corn, in my opinion, resembles wheat pasta the most and has a nice flavor. However, being corn, it's not very healthy for you.

More and more gluten-free pastas are coming on the market every day and in all sorts of combinations. It's always best to look for one that has only a few ingredients, is made primarily out of flours, not starch and with no additives. Look for pastas that have rice flours, quinoa flours; basically, more flour than starch. If there are ingredients on the label you can't pronounce or any nasty E-Numbers, then there might be a better option for you elsewhere.

Supermarkets are great at stocking dried pasta packets and one of my favorite brands is Barilla™. However, if you spend just a little more money, you might find a better option at your local farmers market, or independent grocery store. In

Australia, there is a small retail chain store called IGA. It pales in comparison to the larger stores around the world, but in each region, they stock small boutique products. In my local IGA store I can buy freshly made organic gluten-free pasta, something I can't get at a large chain store.

Once you have nailed down your favorites, I recommend buying a few packets of each and storing them in the cupboard or fridge as it's very frustrating when you run out of something mid-cooking. You might find it's just not that easy anymore to run to the local shop and grab a replacement.

It might take you a little time in the initial stages to figure out your best go-to options, but once you have them, shopping, cooking, and life will become easier.

Chapter 16

To Oat
or Not to Oat?

That is the question and the answer is *yes*…and *no*!

Oats do not contain the same gluten protein found in wheat. Rather, it contains a protein called *avenin sativa* or *avenin* for short. Some celiacs may have an intolerance to this protein and some may not. A very minute percentage of celiacs (less than 10%) can react to the avenin protein in oats, experiencing the same immune response as gluten. Oats, being part of the grain family, contain high levels of those nasty lectins, which also may or may not cause issues for some people.

The best way to help yourself heal is to avoid oats altogether for a while until your body has regenerated its villi, then introduce it slowly and get tests done to see if it's triggering your antibodies and once again destroying your villi. Once you have eliminated gluten completely, it will be easier to tell if you have any reactions to oats. When you first detox from gluten, it can be hard to know what's going on in your body; everything can feel out of balance.

The real issue with oats is cross contamination. Traditionally, oats are grown in the same field areas as wheat. Cross winds and harvesting machines can cause cross contamination, and oats are generally processed in facilities that also process wheat. Is it safe to just buy normal oats off the shelf and eat them? No.

When you're ready to introduce oats again, you will want to look for organic oats as a start but also oats that adhere to a strict contamination-free policy. These are grown in their own fields, harvested and processed separately, and should be from reputable sources. You will want to look for a gluten-free certified brand of oats. Be sure to read their contamination statements. I like to use **Bob's™ Red Mill brand of Gluten Free Oats** which you can buy on **Amazon**, or **iHerb.com**

I used to be a massive porridge eater and I loved making my own granola bars, but I adopted an oat-free diet in the early days. It was hard at first and took some time to adjust but with everything that was going on, I really did not want to take the chance. Since having healed from gluten completely, I took on an oat challenge to see if I was one of the unlucky ones who would react to the avenin. I'm pleased to say I did not react to oats. This news was exciting; I felt like there was one less thing to worry about. However, after spending the first couple of years avoiding oats to heal, I have now found that I don't *want* them like I used to.

When should you consider it? Everyone is different about how they live their gluten-free life and as much as I want to give a recommendation here, I'm erring on the side of caution as I am not a doctor and can't really say. However, common sense to me would be to do a little audit on your health and your diet, and speak to your doctor (or specialist) about when would be a good time.

Because I had regular blood tests every 3 months for a year to check my levels and a follow up biopsy that showed my villi had regenerated, I did this challenge almost two years after diagnosis once I knew I was almost certainly back to normal.

I like oats in porridge on a cold winter's morning and sometimes I'll include them in making my own granola to go with my coconut yogurt, but mainly I mill them into a flour and include it in my sourdough bread recipes. I don't rely on oats the way I once did and eat them sparingly.

If you are gluten-intolerant, you may find that this chapter about oats does not really apply to you unless you are wanting to avoid grains, but if you are celiac, would you take on the oat challenge? If you are one of the lucky ones, would you love to be able to eat oats again?

Chapter 17

The Funny
History of Food Advertising

*D*o you believe everything you see on TV *or* read in magazines? Do you think that drinking Blatz Beer in 1855 while pregnant and breastfeeding was good for your baby, just because the company said, *"The malt in beer supplies nourishing qualities that are essential at this time?"*

The history of food advertising is one of the funniest things to see today, but was it back then? What was the source of information when there was no internet and televisions only graced the homes of the wealthy? How much information do you think your grandparents or great-grandparents had access to, the *right* information, and from which sources? How could you trust a doctor in the 1950s when they promoted cigarettes? How can you trust a doctor today for nutritional advice when they study medicine and not nutrition?

I found an advertisement for Wheatena™ Cereal that was published in a local paper sometime around the early 1900s with a headline *"Worth A Million Pound – Are they gaining or losing weight?"* It reads:

"One out of every three school children is under-weight, therefore under-nourished. The chief cause - doctors say - is improper diet. Too much super-refined foods! Too little natural foods that build strong, sturdy bodies and sound robust health. That's why Doctors today so strongly urge hot all-wheat cereal with milk. It supplies - in the proportions - the 16 vital food elements needed for health, for strength, for energy and for growth. Wheatena is the cereal that brings you - at no extra cost- the priceless food materials that nature packs into the nut-brown wheat kernel."

How do you argue with an advertisement like this in your local paper when that is your only means of access to information?

It seemed women started paying attention to their weight and dieting started to become a thing. Companies back then probably didn't want to lose out on sales because housewives were not purchasing their products anymore. So, what better way to make sure you're capturing all consumer markets than with an advertisement that was posted in the mid 1950s with a headline "*If you're dieting to lose weight.*" It reads:

> *"Whether you are trying to reduce safely or trying to feed your family well and economically, this new knowledge can help you. Besides food energy, there are five other nutrients in modern enriched bread and all the delicious foods made from flour. From no other source can you get these nutrients so inexpensively and so temptingly, day after day. Buy enriched bread and other baked foods; use enriched flour always...for 6-way nourishment!" "The nutritional statements in this advertisement are acceptable to the Council on Foods and Nutrition of the American Medical Association."*

Fast forward to the late 1960s and advertisements are appealing to a younger audience too. In 1968 a full-page advertisement for Wonderbread™ was in a magazine with a sexy-looking woman holding a white bread sandwich out to the reader. It reads:

> *"Are you the kind of girl boys fall in love with at the drop of your false lashes? Is your mailbox overflowing with torrid love letters? Say you play the dating game to win. But don't forget, catching his eye is one thing; keeping it's another. Be a little sneaky. Remember, boys love to eat. And they love Wonder sandwiches, too. So get Wonder going for you."*

Looking back at these advertisements really made me think about food advertising, the limited access to information, and how previous generations were guided on what were the right foods to eat. *Also, I really, really wanted to include pictures for these ads—they look absolutely hilarious—but I'm not allowed to because of copyright infringements.*

I know that when I was younger, I certainly ate cereals, breads, and all sorts of wheat-related items. It was simply what we ate. My childhood diet was not filled with kale, quinoa, and cacao. It *was* Kellogg's Nutri-grain™ for breakfast and it was white bread for lunch and pasta for dinner.

My parents didn't know back then that this food was unhealthy and killing me slowly from the inside out. How could they? These were pre-internet days, and access to information was limited. There was one doctor in the local town nearby and he didn't know much about nutrition, allergies, or auto-immune diseases.

I thoroughly believe we are at a turning point in food history and are in the center of the *age of information* as free access to information has never been easier. There are no more excuses or reasons preventing the majority of people from learning about food, nutrition, or their health. Here are a few examples of just how easy it is for us to learn:

- I just recently attended a 'Gluten-free Food Expo' which was unheard of years ago.

- I have a Thermomix® that beams healthy recipes from cyberspace to the machine itself in my kitchen.

- I can Google just about anything, attend webinars, and research articles from my phone in bed.

- I can now video chat with a specialist in any country and email some of the best clinics in the world for information.

- I can see first-hand through the National Centre for Biotechnology and Information the latest research papers on celiac disease.

- Book stores are flooded with books on diseases and allergies and if I don't feel like going to a book store, I can order anything from Amazon and have it delivered in days.

- Libraries are constantly buying similar books to mainstream bookstores and are flooded with a range of health topics. I actually found one library to contain more books on health than the local book shop. The best part…it's free to learn. You don't have to purchase a book.

- When I don't have time to read, I can listen to an audiobook while driving.

My point to all of this is that, for many people, there is no excuse to be ignorant about their health, their diet, or the available options. The hard part now is that we are being bombarded with *so* much information that we have to sift through it all to find out what's true and what's not true. I can look up a question on the internet today, such as *"Is gluten bad for you?"* and have a 50/50 response for yes and no.

With the mass availability of information, more people like myself are getting educated, and as much as that is a good thing, it can also make things difficult for others to discern who and what to believe. For example, I have researched some of the world's specialists and found that saturated fat *does not* cause heart disease, yet my television news station has a doctor who is also a nutritionist featured regularly saying that *it does*?

If you are presented with something on TV and it's in your face randomly on the 7 o' clock news, one would suppose you would believe it, right? But how do you know it's true? How do you know what they are presenting to you is the correct information unless you have researched other specialists to find out other studies? That's hard work and most people don't want to do it. Even today, what looks like an unbiased news reporter article on TV, is actually a cleverly designed paid advertisement and most people are none the wiser.

Facebook groups are a great way to get some guidance and learn about what others are going through, but not everyone is an expert. I have seen comments to a person's post that I know are simply not correct. I sometimes intervene with the relevant research or link to the correct information, but this usually doesn't go down too well. People don't like to be corrected in public as a general rule. Neither am I an expert; I'm just somebody who has studied the guts out of celiac disease. Do I know everything? No. Does it mean you should believe every word I say? No. But you should take the information I have gathered, cross check it against the proper resources, and apply what *you think* is best for *you*.

A great idea is to build your own resource library of trusted authorities. I've listed just a few of my trusted mentors below. These are the people I have learned from and continue to learn from; they are the world leaders on inflammation and celiac disease.

- **Dr. Tom O'Bryan.** A global leader in functional medicine and celiac disease expert. (www.thedr.com)

- **Dr. David Perlmutter.** A renowned neurologist who's an expert in gluten issues, brain health, nutrition, and preventing neurodegenerative disorders. (www.drperlmutter.com)

- **Dr. Peter Green**. A gastroenterologist and professor of clinical medicine. He is also the director of the Celiac Disease Center at Columbia University. (https://celiacdiseasecenter.columbia.edu)

- **Dr. Alejandro Junger**. An eastern medicine specialist, cardiologist, and founder of The Clean Program. (www.thecleanprogram.com)

- **Brenda Watson**. Clinical nutritionist, author, and PBS-TV health educator. (www.brendawatson.com)

- **Dr. Leo Galland.** World leader in integrated medicine and founder of Functional Medicine. (www.drgalland.com)

- **Dr. Peter Osborne.** World leader in functional medicine and Celiac Disease. (www. https://drpeterosborne.com)

Chapter 18

Survival Tools
for the New World

I call it a new world because for me it literally was. The world of happy go-lucky, eat-on-the-fly, and the care-free attitude I had was gone. I had to learn to eat differently and live differently. This was a lifelong commitment of change and I could either choose to let it get the best of me *or* create a new world that I could live within.

- I didn't want to live a life that was culinarily restricted, so I had to learn how to prep food in advance, in a totally different way and with ingredients I had not heard of before.

- I couldn't just order something random to eat at a hawker food stand in Hong Kong anymore, so I had to learn to communicate my stupid disease, sometimes to those who didn't speak English, when I traveled.

- I didn't want to miss dining out with my friends and family, so I had to learn to make eating out an easier and a hassle-free experience.

- Going gluten-free can sometimes feel like an emotional roller coaster, so I had to learn to deal with new emotions like want-but-can't-have.

- It's one thing thinking you can just eat gluten-free, but it's another thing to learn to create a gluten-free environment. Here, I share my honest thoughts on how strict I am around cross contamination.

The following chapters are my tips, hints, and ideas that I want to share with you, on how I've dealt with the topics above.

Understanding cross contamination

Cross contamination and how to deal with it is pretty serious food for thought. Knowing it only takes something as small as 1/70th of a piece of bread (50 milligrams) to start destroying villi is sobering. There's a spotlight on cross contamination due to the concerns of celiac disease patients not fully healing and developing more health issues. It's an ongoing issue to deal with whether at home, at work, eating out, or even buying prepared meals labeled gluten-free.

Contamination in the home

Cross contamination can lurk at home, not only in food but dish towels, rags, sponges, utensils, and food prep equipment like waffle irons and toasters.

To handle it most effectively, first decide if you are in a family where you need to have gluten in the home. If so, then the standard recommendation at home is to have a separate toaster, cooking utensils, and cutting boards. For cleaning the kitchen clean, you might want to buy a dedicated set of colored sponges that are only used for non-gluten-free meals. The use of paper towels is exceptional at preventing cross contamination but does come at a tax to nature. Use wraps and labeled snap lock bags to separate meals. One of the big-ticket items is flour, so it is a good idea to keep wheat flour in a separate cupboard and labeled clearly where there is a less likely risk of a mix up. Perhaps having discussions and teaching sessions with your family members about cross contamination will help or are they able to support you and eat mostly what you eat?

Contamination when dining out

Where you're dining out will dictate the level of risk. Are you eating at a certified celiac-friendly restaurant or are you eating at Taco Bell™? Some restaurants offer many gluten-free meals but cannot offer a gluten-free kitchen, meaning other gluten-containing meals are still being prepared there. It will come down to talking to the restaurant to determine what their practices are when handling meals. Are they well versed in gluten-free and take all best efforts to do the right thing, or are they a little haphazard about it? Do they clearly label their meals GF or is there no labeling at all? I cover more about dining out in the chapter **How to eat out and not die...*from the aftermath*** but there is still a risk to keep in the back of your mind.

Contamination of packaged goods

There is a risk, albeit very small, even when buying packaged food. There is an organization called **Gluten Free Watchdog** which provides unbiased reporting and state-of-the-art gluten-free food testing data for consumers on packaged foods. Many times, I've seen them release emails about re-called gluten-free products or products with misleading labels.

But what does this all mean for us? It means we have to learn what we are willing and not willing to accept, and what is achievable to integrate into our life and how far are we willing to take it. For some, a single crumb can cause upset. According to reports, however, 50 milligrams of gluten is what it takes to initiate the auto-immune response; this is more than a single crumb. This is not to say that hyper-sensitive people don't react in some way.

For the first 6 to 12 months after diagnosis, I was so strict on the subject of cross-contamination, especially in my own home, that I was stressing myself out trying to adhere to all the rules. I read all the books and did what they all said: used a different toaster, had separate utensils and chopping boards. But I was struggling to manage this and not only was it taking up space in my small kitchen, it was taking up space in my mind. I think of myself as lucky and don't react to a single crumb of gluten, but I still tried to follow all the rules.

My husband once said to me that I was worrying so much about cross contamination everywhere that I was probably doing my body more harm than good; I was probably creating more inflammation from the stress of trying to follow so many rules. And he was right! Stress is one of the worst things you can do to your body and it wreaks havoc anywhere it can, in any form. So, what was going to be worse? A tiny piece of wheat crumb in the toaster or the stress and arguments about it in the first place? I also don't have a wheat allergy and know that one tiny crumb does not equate to 50 milligrams of gluten so I'm not going to fuss over it. For others though, this is a different story.

I am very lucky that my husband chose to go gluten-free with me. We don't have any children and he was happy to eat all the alternatives but requested his one vice of bread. We chatted about cross contamination from the bread but he made a deal to be diligent, wash everything properly, and not double dip his knife in the butter.

As much as this disease is serious, most of us with celiac disease (wheat allergy excluded) don't go into anaphylactic shock and die on the spot. I needed to keep reminding myself of this. I needed to feel like I was still living life, rather than living in a bubble of segregation and fear.

Before I was diagnosed celiac, I remember a friend, Ben, who has a nut allergy, telling me about a reaction he had at work. Not knowing much about nut allergies and what really happens, I listened intently.

 One day at work, the poor guy was given something with nuts in it and was going into cardiac arrest right there and then on the floor. Ben worked with my husband and had tried to scream out to him off in the distance for help but his throat constricted and his heart slowed down. From where my husband was standing, he couldn't hear what Ben was saying but saw him collapse to the ground and put two and two together. My husband sprinted to Ben's work bag, grabbed his EpiPen® and darted back as fast as his feet could carry him. At this point Ben was unconscious on the ground. My husband jabbed him right in the thigh. Sure enough, it revived him, got his airway open, and off to hospital he went.

The point of my story is this: if you do your best to go gluten-free, a little bit of accidental exposure won't kill you. Yes, you will get sick. Yes, you will feel crappy for days. Yes, repeated crumb incidents might cause damage to your villi and long term health and even though that is serious, keep in mind you won't die on the spot. Your gut can repair; it has an amazing ability to regenerate very quickly within a matter of days! I'm not going to judge anyone on their practices of how they live their life around gluten, but I do want to say, try not to stress yourself out about it. I did in the beginning, a lot, and it was tiring. Be mindful, be diligent, learn how to handle cross contamination in different situations but still live life.

Contamination mishap learning curve

I thought that you needed to eat gluten to get sick; turns out, you can breathe it in too. When visiting a friend, I made her beef stroganoff and used traditional wheat flour to coat the beef. I spooned the flour into a bag with the beef and shook it around, opened it up and tipped the beef out into the hot pan, then repeated the process two more times. Halfway through cooking her meal, I started to get bloated and tired. My stomach blew out to looking like I was nine months pregnant and I had instant narcolepsy.

I left the kitchen, fell onto the couch clutching my stomach, broke out in a heavy sweat, and passed out for hours. I woke and felt unwell for the next day or so, but before you knew it, I was back up and running again. I learned two lessons here: one was that a bit of accidental gluten exposure won't kill me; and two was don't ever cook with wheat flour again, even for someone else.

It's all about the prep

One thing I learned very quickly is that preparation is the key to prevent getting *fangry* (f*king angry-hungry) .

I can no longer travel at a moment's notice to somewhere I haven't been and think I'll be able to find something to eat along the way. I've tried that and it was very frustrating, which resulted in a little starvation and getting *fangry*.

I travel around a lot for my work and I can tell you that in Australia the highway gas station stops usually don't cater to people like us. Sometimes the best I could find was an apple. How unsatisfying! I want my journeys locally and abroad to be filled with more choice than an apple!

On one work trip, I called into a small bakery as it said on their website that they had gluten-free salads. But when I arrived and saw baguettes sitting right on top of them I walked away, hungry and disappointed. Learning that I needed to be more proactive in my preparation for work-life, I now take the following steps.

- I always keep protein bars in my handbag for those hunger pangs when I just can't find anything on the run.

- I keep my favorite bread in the freezer at work and some nut spread in the fridge, so if I get stuck one day and don't have time to pack lunch, there is a back-up ready and waiting.

- I also have organic *heat and serve* curries that sit in the drawer of my desk. I'm not one for many products like this, as I believe fresh is best, but this particular curry is additive free, healthy, and used only in emergency situations. This is a great option if you only have access to a microwave.

- I even have a bottle of tamari sauce stashed under the seat of my car so that, if I'm driving around and I see a quick take away sushi shop, I've got my dipping sauce ready to go. Most sushi shops don't sell GF soy sauce.

(Note: most good sushi restaurants have a range of gluten-free sushi rolls, however some establishments put flour in the rice mixture or regular soy sauce in the tuna mixtures, so it always pays to check).

Sometimes my husband and I like to have date nights at home. They previously consisted of bread, cured meats, dumplings (aka potstickers), cheese, etc. Now that I can no longer eat half of those yummy snack items, I needed to find alternatives. To accompany our olives, cheese, and nitrate-free prosciutto, I now make crumbed chicken nuggets, coconut crumbed prawns, arancini balls, and miniature quiches; I keep them in the freezer. The freezer went from storing ice and beer to storing all sorts of yummy ready-to-go snacks, including raw berry cheesecake deserts.

When eating meals at home, I soon realized that I couldn't whip up something last minute for lunch or dinner. It often would be missing some ingredients if I hadn't pre-planned the meal. By the time I'd driven to a shop to get the right ingredients, I was pretty *hangry* and hating my disease because I couldn't just grab my husband's wheat bread and slather it with peanut butter to get me out of trouble until I could get to the store. So now, I always make sure to buy items in bulk or shop more regularly.

Eggs became my best friend. I probably eat on average two eggs a day. They contain fantastic healthy fats, protein, and are just downright yummy. I know they don't suit everyone but for me, they are a balanced blend of nutrients and easy to come by, so they're great to have on hand. Breakfast in a rush is simply two scrambled eggs with some avocado. For snacks, I have boiled eggs in the fridge ready for a quick and filling bite to eat.

After getting stuck for food a few times at home, I now stock up on all sorts of strange and wonderful healthy GF alternatives like quinoa crackers, paleo bread, brown rice pasta twirls, falafel mix, konjac noodles, nut butters, and tuna. I can easily throw something together with these basics. Once I began to include these little new odd items in my regular shopping routine, my cupboards were always well stocked right when I needed it, thus eliminating the *fangry* feeling and the emotional tantrum that followed.

For in-between meal snacks, I usually prepare a large batch of protein/energy bars and keep them in the fridge for a week or two. Mixed nuts became a regular part of my diet. A handful of nuts on the go is just enough to keep the hunger pangs down until mealtime.

When driving to visit family, I will usually pack an Esky© with some snacks, bread for breakfast, eggs, and a packet of my favorite GF pasta. Just a few basics to get by when I arrive or until I get to the store. I'll also order things online and have it delivered there ahead of time.

When I would attend dinner gatherings with friends after I was first diagnosed, I used to get so upset and frustrated with myself and this stupid disease because I could not eat all that wonderful food. Shortly after learning how to live with my diagnosis, I went to a hen's party for my close friend and the table was full of lovely snack items that I could not eat except for some cheese and grapes. But this time, rather than getting upset and going hungry, I had my little bag of treats in my handbag, crackers being one of them. I quietly put the cheese on top of my own crackers when no one was looking and joined the conversations.

When I was diagnosed, I was so ashamed of my disease and embarrassed that I was no longer the care-free food enthusiast I once was. I always hated girls who had to make a fuss over their so-called *diet restrictions* and never wanted to be seen in this category. I used to hover around food tables pretending to eat so no one saw that I was *not* really eating. This avoided the explanation, *"Oh I can't have that, I have celiac disease."* Sometimes it was just nicer to blend in without having to be the center of attention with what's touted as a trendy food allergy or have the host feel uneasy.

However, fast forward to today (four years later) and how I manage eating out with friends is a different story. Yes, I'll still pack crackers in my handbag to put with cheese, but I no longer do it in secret. I just go about my business and if someone asks, I'll gladly explain to them. When I first started doing this, I was surprised to find out just how many other people have diet restrictions, took it seriously and not like a trendy weight loss method. I even learned some tips and tricks from others, like keeping miniature sauce and dressing satchels in my handbag to put with salads and other items I could eat. I also realized that with the increasing prevalence of celiac disease, the more people I can educate about it the better. Someone knows someone with celiac disease or a gluten sensitivity. Wouldn't the world be a bit nicer for that sufferer if their friend or colleague understood more about it?

The key takeaway from these stories is that being prepared is key to an easier journey with your diagnosis. Like everything, prep takes practice and soon, hopefully, it will form part of your regular routine.

Key preparation points:

- Keep snack bars in your handbag or man-bag.

- If you frequently visit family or friends, leave a box of snack bars, crackers, or anything you like with them so that it's there for when you visit.

- Order food online and have it sent to your destination.

- Keep emergency food items at work in the fridge, cupboard, or your desk area.

- Research some great freezer recipes and cook in batches ahead of time for entertaining.

- Buy your staples in bulk; don't buy one packet of GF pasta, buy three.

- When dining at group gatherings with friends, talk to the host if the occasion fits and find out what might be safe for you to eat, eat beforehand, or pack a few crackers or something you know you will be able to put with something else on offer.

How to eat out and not die...*from the aftermath*

Get used to the idea very quickly that you're going to be that annoying customer at a restaurant that has to ask, *"Can you make this gluten-free?"* or *"Excuse me, but are you sure this is gluten-free?"*

Before my diagnosis I was so proud that I was such an easy-going eater, especially when dining out with my husband or friends. I remember being out at dinner and one friend said at our Japanese banquet, *"Excuse me, please don't add sodium."* I loved her to bits but geez she was a pain in the ass acting all high-and-mighty over some salt. Why couldn't she ask for *less salt* rather than having to say *sodium*. Who does that?

Another friend at the table said, *"Oh, I can't have that, gluten doesn't work well with me."* I thought to myself, *"Geez people, if you're not going to die, stop making such a fuss here in front of everyone and just suck it up."*

My husband leaned over to me at that point and whispered in my ear, *"Oh honey I'm so glad you're not high maintenance like that!"*

Now, I have egg on my face. I *am* one of *those* people.

I'm trying my hardest to embrace it, but I do struggle from time to time. I'm very fortunate to have such a supportive husband even though now I'm high maintenance. When we are out, my husband makes a joke in his comical voice to the waitstaff saying, *"She's a little special and doesn't get out very often. Do you have anything gluten-free? She has a disease!"*

At this point, the waitstaff is laughing, and along with me having a sheepish shy grin, the ice is broken. This is now our new little routine when we go out.

Tales of dining-out mishaps

The first few times eating out, I inquired about some meals to double check if it was going to be gluten-free and the response was, yes they were gluten-free. Yet I was glutened on more than one occasion. I became pissed off and very wary of eating out, so I hid within the confines of my home kitchen until the pissed-off wore off.

I learned pretty quickly to use my own judgement to decide if a meal would contain gluten or not based on the ingredients. I learned not to rely on the word of the wait staff, especially when they sounded slightly vague. Body language also plays an important role in determining if someone really knows enough to confidently answer. There have been many times where I would ask, *"If I removed the bun from this chicken burger, would it then ensure that the meal will be gluten-free?"* and the response was, *"Eh, yeah...sure."* Based on that reaction, I would order something else.

On another occasion, I saw a burger that had a gluten-free bun option. But knowing that sometimes breadcrumbs could be added to meat patties, I asked the wait staff, *"Does this meat patty contain any breadcrumbs? I'm celiac and can't take the risk."* She went to ask the cook in the kitchen and his repose was, *"Yes, we do use just a little bit of breadcrumbs, so it should be ok!"* What the ...? I thought. No, it's not ok for just a little bit. Celiacs cannot ever have *just* a little bit! So, another tip, don't ever assume that burger patties are free from breadcrumbs. At first, I was so annoyed when I heard that response but then again, we can't assume everyone including chefs know as much about gluten as we do. I knew nothing about gluten before I was diagnosed.

On the flip side, I have had some wonderful experiences also. I came across one restaurant that was very informed when I asked if I could have the baked eggs without any bread and checked if there was anything else in the mixture of the beans that would contain gluten, just to be certain. The young woman said to me, *"Oh, are you celiac?"*

I was a little taken aback at her inquiry. I replied, *"Yes, and newly diagnosed, too. So, I'm sorry for questioning the food."* She said she had a friend who was celiac and understood all about it. Then she proceeded to explain that she had a small kitchen and couldn't really guarantee there would not be any cross contamination but would do her absolute best to make sure the meal was free of any gluten ingredients. I smiled and felt a wave of relief, understanding, and acceptance from this woman. She offered to exchange the bread to a gluten-free quinoa potato patty instead at no charge. I was shocked and happy all at the same time. When the food came it was absolutely delicious. I didn't get sick and needless to say I put that restaurant on my favorites list.

It's not too difficult for food establishments to let us know whether or not they are equipped to handle food for celiacs. There is a difference between serving gluten-free food and having a celiac-friendly environment in which the food is prepped and free of contamination.

Whilst many restaurants offer a range of gluten-free meals, the establishment themselves may not contaminate-free. Even though a meal might have gluten-free ingredients, you need to also trust the preparation method will be ok. You can do this by stating to the server that you have celiac disease and are highly sensitive to gluten. This will usually prompt them to explain their situation for handling food or mark it down on the order so the chefs in the kitchen can see. They might explain in a similar method above—they cannot guarantee contaminate-free—or they might tell you that they are fully equipped and trained to handle your food or they might tell you that to be safe, you should eat somewhere else. Some establishments put a disclaimer at the bottom of their menu such as, *"Our kitchen is not contaminate-free of major allergens. While every effort is made to provide you with your requested meal, please keep in mind that our deep fryer and grills are shared. Please notify your server if you have an allergen and we will take every effort we can but cannot guarantee your meal to be 100% allergen free."*

At the end of the day, I don't expect establishments to fully cater to me but knowing how they handle food lets *me* make a judgement as to whether or not I'll dine there.

Another tale of a dining out mishap involved forgetting a technical name for wheat. You really need to understand the other names of wheat so you don't get caught out unaware. They can be a mouthful and easy to forget. Sometimes when you're reading a menu, establishments use so many fancy words they all just blur. I hadn't really heard of this one much before, and I didn't have my little cheat sheets in my handbag. Here's how it happened.

I was in LA with my friend, dining at a fine Italian restaurant in Manhattan Beach before I had to jump on a plane back to Australia. We sat at the bar, ordered our French Oak Vanilla Tannin Bordeaux while perusing the menu. In our usual style, we wanted to try a little bit of everything, so we ordered several half-size meals to share. Now, my friend is not celiac but she is gluten-sensitive so we were both looking out for each other on what to order. Once satisfied with our in-depth discussion on desire and accompaniments, we ordered the following:

- **Bresaola:** *Aged air-dried beef topped with tomato, rucola and aged balsamic.*

- **Prosciutto e mousse di Parmigiano:** *Imported artisan cured grand reserve prosciutto served with parmesan cheese mousse*

- **Insalata Mista:** *Mixed leaves with cucumber, farro, and olives tossed in a red wine vinegar*

We actually ordered way more food than this, but this will give you an idea.

When the tall, dark, and handsome waiter looking back at me with *those* eyes came to take our order, I stuttered that I was celiac and if he would make a note on the order so it was known in the kitchen to be careful. The menu did not mention if any meals were gluten-free, but by this point, I thought I was pretty good at determining if a meal contained gluten or not without having to ask and make a big fuss. We thought we'd chosen well in that instance. *But did we?*

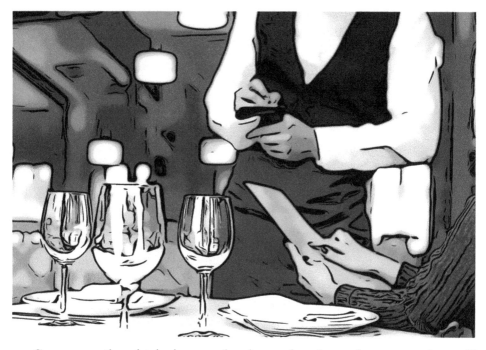

Can you see the mistake in my order above where I was about to get glutened? Mr. Waiter leaned over the bar and pointed to the Insalata Mista on the menu and said in that smoky baritone voice, *"Bella, are youa sure you wanta orda thisa meal? Tis no gluten-freeo!"*

I blinked twice and replied in my Aussie accent, *"Really? How come?"*

He pointed to the word *farro* on the description of the meal and said, *"This isa wheata!"*

I looked like a stunned mullet for a brief moment and was shocked at my stupidity. I'd just totally embarrassed myself not knowing a fancy word for a variety of wheat in a fancy restaurant. Once I got over my ego embarrassment a wave of relief went through me and I was happy that he knew his menu well enough to pick that up. Needless to say, we didn't have the salad and left him a generous tip.

There are no guarantees

Still to this day, even though I might take every precaution when ordering, eating out is a gamble. I recently went to one of my favorite burger joints that caters to celiacs and the food is safe to eat, but perhaps this day they had new staff. I went through the same process of ordering, received my meal, and ate it like a hungry vulture, enjoying every bite. I finished my meal with satisfaction and went on to complete my grocery shopping. *Tip: Never go grocery shopping when you're hungry.*

About 30 minutes passed and all of a sudden the gurgling stomach started, the cramping started, the yawns started. *Oh no, not here pleeeassseeee!* I pleaded to my two anal sphincters to work with me and stay firmly shut like a dolphin's ass. *Anywhere but a shopping center,* I thought.

I dumped my trolley full of groceries and my walk quickly became a run as I whizzed past shoppers to the public toilets. I pushed past an old lady *(so sorry!)* and damn near kicked the door into the cubicle, head butted it shut behind me while my hands were busy tearing my pants off and...*Ka-boom!*

After what felt like an hour of hot and cold sweats, shivers, stomach pains, and a lot of noise, I emerged from Chernobyl and stumbled back to my car like a drunken idiot, to go home where I would sleep it off for the next day. So, even sometimes your most trusted restaurants can have slip ups every now and again.

Turns out just because I was asymptomatic when I was eating gluten before diagnosis, doesn't mean I stayed that way after detoxing from gluten. I had turned into a human gluten detector, trace amounts or gluten (or accidentally inhaling it) induces the worst reactions now, whereas this never used to be the case. I'm not sure if this is the case for all Asymptomatic but I would really like to know.

Here are my tips to avoid a nuclear catastrophe

1. Keep a diary

When eating out, keep a journal of the good places you go that worked out well. I like to keep a little section on my phone where I take a picture of the menu and the meal so I can remember easily for next time. One of the editors of this book uses a Google Maps system where she 'stars' a favorite place from a top-notch experience or an accredited place so she can see geographically what's nearby. What a great idea, and I thought I was a geek, ha ha.

2. Phone ahead

If you're going to meet friends out, get online and look at the menu first. If it's not labeled clearly enough for you, phone ahead and work out a meal that you can order. Then, when you arrive, you can pretend you're browsing through the menu then order at the same time as everyone else. This way, ordering is hassle-free and you avoid feeling like you're making a scene by asking too many questions. I hated doing this at first but it's easier to hide behind a phone and ask all the questions you want, as you can't see the other person's body language or frustration.

Phoning ahead sometimes has its surprises. I was back in Las Vegas and this was the first trip after being diagnosed. I was trying to Google where I could eat, as all my usual places had heavily gluten-filled menus. I wanted *so* much to go back to the Caesars Palace buffet. For some reason, I tend to suffer from gluttony when in Vegas. There are just so many food options.

All of a sudden, my wishes were answered. Just as I was thinking about a buffet and drooling like Homer Simpson, I read somewhere randomly that if you phone ahead to Caesars and let them know you have an allergy, they will send one of the chefs or representatives out to meet with you and walk you through on what you can and can't have. You didn't have to ask me twice if I wanted to go and dear hubby didn't get a choice in the matter. I was on the phone making a reservation for that very night.

Sure enough, as the forum said, a waiter came out from the kitchen to confirm that I was celiac and then walked with me from one end of the mile-long buffet to the other, pointing to each and every dish and advising me what was safe and not safe for me to eat. Even when it came to the desert bar, he pointed at over half a dozen items I *could* eat. I was so excited, I seriously felt like I had my own personal food guide for the evening. So, phoning ahead sometimes does have its advantages.

3.   How to Survive Functions & Conventions

If you get stuck at a function or a convention, while everyone is busy mingling before the sit-down, quickly excuse yourself to the bathroom but divert to one of the staff and check what's being served. If there is nothing you can have, tell the chef you're celiac. They usually accommodate for this quite easily. Ask them to deliver your meal at the same time as everyone else's and tell them what you look like. This way, if all goes well, your meal arrives without fuss.

I did not know you could do this, so the first time I went to a function, I looked like an idiot.

Not long after being diagnosed, we had to attend a function. We all sat down in our black-tie outfits and I looked at the menu and had a choice of gluten, gluten, *and* gluten. I sat a little uneasily for a while thinking, *What am I going to do?*

First, they delivered the side of bread rolls, which I politely pretended I didn't notice by being too busy sipping on my champagne and making small talk with the other guests. Then came the main meal. I casually ate the bit of untainted potato off the side of the plate, then messed up my food a little to make it look like I'd attempted to eat, then gently pushed the plate back to say I was finished.

Again, I continued with the chatter and champagne. I thought I was off the hook until the person to one side of me noticed I hadn't eaten much and caught my odd glance at the food. I just grinned and said, *"I had a late lunch at work"* but then my idiot husband blurted out, *"She's got celiac disease!"*

Argh, bloody bastard, I thought as I slapped my head with my hand and slid into my seat with embarrassment. It's one thing doing that at a cafe, but at a gala function, really?

Now everyone was questioning me, making it a big deal. Now, I felt like I was one of *those* people. I had people trying to offer me their food, which wasn't helping the situation, and then one of the table guests went up and got a waitress and said: *"She has celiac disease, can you make her something else to eat?"* At this point, I just wanted to run and hide in the bathroom.

Seeing my discomfort, one of the other ladies leaned over and quietly told me she was a vegan and everything on the menu was meat. Yet, I hadn't noticed anything different while she was eating. She blended in so seamlessly. I actually didn't think such a large organization would cater to anything other than what was booked for the menu, so I was relieved to know otherwise. She then proceeded to tell me how to navigate these situations.

4. Double check the menu

Double check your menu items if they look suspect. Don't trust the menu on its own. I ordered a bacon, egg, and cheese roll one day and it was clearly labeled gluten-free, but when it came out, I noticed it had BBQ sauce on it, which I used to love. I had to stop a moment and think. Then I asked the waitress about the sauce as it wasn't listed on the menu. I asked the chef to check that particular sauce brand and sure enough, they returned to remove my meal. The sauce had gluten in it.

5. Get out of your comfort zone

I took my husband out for a birthday lunch to a lavish floating seafood restaurant. In my head I'm thinking, *"Surely at least I can order grilled fish and salad and be in the clear."* When we arrived, he saw the seafood tower on the menu and gave me that look of, *"Gee I want this but know you can't have it."* Not wanting to disappoint him, I put my big girl pants on and pulled the waiter over and whispered to him, *"Hey, I love the sound of this seafood tower, but I have celiac disease. Is there anything we can substitute to make it ok for me to eat?"*

I probably spoke a little too fast and too strong as I was worried I'd chicken out mid-sentence. But it worked. The waiter replied, *"Yes ma'am, we can swap the deep-fried shrimp for some BBQ shrimp, add in some extra oysters, grill the fish instead, and swap out the fried calamari for seared salt and pepper calamari. We will give you some extra gluten-free dressings on the side and fry your chips in a dedicated fryer that has not come in contact with gluten. Oh, and the lobster, fruit, and salads are perfectly safe to eat."*

I didn't know if I was falling off my chair or having an orgasm. After a little shuffle to regain my senses, I confidently looked back and said, *"That's great. We'll have all that and a bottle of your finest Pinot Gris, please!"*

My husband was lost for words at my poised assertiveness and then began to giggle at me as I apparently had a look of '*Little Miss Confident*' across my face.

Pizza. Boy, did I miss pizza. I'm not a fan of the usual chain stores and I'm sure you can guess why, so I went on the hunt to find a pizza store nearby that could hopefully cater to my whims.

I phoned around and scoured the net to see what I could find. About a 15-minute drive from where I live is a little old rustic Italian joint. I wasn't hopeful, but when the lady on the other end of the phone advised me that they do in fact have gluten-free bases, I was happy to give this place a try. I was even happier when she said they get them in fresh every day from a local supplier, they are cooked on their own trays, and cut on a separate cutting board with their own pizza knife. All the toppings were also gluten-free, so I didn't have to worry about that either. Needless to say, I'm now back on schedule with Friday Pizza Nights. My husband even orders the gluten-free base, as he seems to like it more than the regular one.

So, get out of your comfort zone, call around, scout out, and don't be afraid to ask.

6. Take responsibility for yourself and be understanding.

Not everyone is going to be as educated on gluten as you are, and at the end of the day, you're responsible for what you put in your mouth; no one else.

I've read some books that say email your dietary requirements to a restaurant and ask what you can and cannot eat. I don't know how much I really agree with this, as I think you should take some responsibility and look at the menu ahead of time, work out what you think you might like, and discuss this with the kitchen staff. If you show a food establishment that you are trying to work with them on what you can eat, it will go a lot further in terms of service and respect than if you were to just tell them you're celiac and expect them to come up with options and meals for you.

I know how frustrating it is sometimes when you can't find a place that is safe to eat. In one of my neighborhoods, I went to 3 different cafés in a row looking for food and it was clearly not going to be safe to eat in any of them. I walked away tired, hungry, and really upset with my disease. However, we need to remember that people create restaurants out of a desire to provide the food *they* love to the world. Celiacs are 1% of the population and I don't believe we should expect that all restaurants should specifically cater to us if they don't want to. It's still their food, the way they choose to present it, and we either eat it or not. I get annoyed when hearing about gluten-sensitive people (celiacs included) having an attitude toward restaurants, as if the business should bow down to their intolerances/diseases and cater to them like they are the queen bee. If that's what you want, go find a certified celiac-friendly place to eat or create your own. There are a growing number of soy allergies, dairy allergies, and even anaphylaxis is fatal to almost 1% of the 5% of sufferers in the United States[71]. Put this together with celiac disease and it can make it difficult for restaurants to cater to everyone.

In saying that though, there is no place for rudeness or attitude from an establishment when you are being declined. What I went through when I was first diagnosed with a chef treating me in a racist way? That's just not called for;   there

[71] Turner, P.J., Jerschow, E., Umasunthar, T., Lin, R., Campbell, D.E., and Boyle, R.J. (2017). "Fatal Anaphylaxis: Mortality Rate and Risk Factors". *J Allergy Clin Immunol Pract.*, 5(5):1169-1178. doi:10.1016/j.jaip.2017.06.031

needs to be kindness on both sides. When I dine out at a restaurant that's not fully designed to cater for my disease, I am absolutely humbled that the chefs and wait staff are willing to deviate from the menus they have designed so I can have a nice experience.

7. Don't get your knickers in a bunch

I had a situation where I ordered a burger from the local brewery to take back to work. I asked them to make it gluten-free, as they offered gluten-free alternatives. When I got back to work with the food, I pulled the burger out, picked it up and went to take a bite when I had a stop moment. The bun felt overly *soft* for gluten-free, and it had a light dusting of white stuff over the top. It felt a little too *springy* to the touch for my liking.

I phoned up the restaurant and asked them if it was definitely gluten-free, and sure enough, once the waitress checked with the chef, she apologized and said, *"No it wasn't."* They were apologetic for getting the order wrong and were happy to make another one for me. I was disappointed but couldn't be bothered going back to get another one so I politely declined. One of the women I worked with talked me into going back so I wouldn't get *fangry* later. I think she knew me.

I went back and collected the replacement burger. I could have easily made a big deal and caused a scene over the whole thing, but instead I politely said to them, *"Hey guys, I know mix ups can happen easily and I probably wouldn't be so concerned if it weren't for the fact that I have celiac disease. Do you think it will be ok in the future to continue to order this?"* They assured me it was gluten-free, gave me some extra hot chips to go with it, and apologized again. They were really trying to make up for it.

In the end, I ate the burger, which was a Philly Cheese Steak Burger. It had smoked brisket with roasted red pepper, confit onion, American cheddar, capsicum jam, and truffle aioli. Needless to say, I didn't get sick at all and it was probably one of the most amazing burgers I have ever eaten.

I thoroughly believe that being courteous to people, even when you need to discuss something as serious as this mistake, goes a lot further than being mean. I phrased my serious concern as a polite question and my relationship with this establishment is even better now. They know me like a local and they probably take more care for other allergy meals because they don't have a bad taste in their mouth from some stuck-up bitch throwing a tantrum.

Go-to take-out

There is still hope if you're careful! Below is a list of navigating take-out food in gluten-free style.

- **Indian**

Typically, Indian curries are made with coconut milk, cashews, yogurt, chickpea flour, and lots of spices rather than wheat-based starch. Poppadum—the thin, crisp, round flatbread served in restaurants—is usually made with rice and lentil flour but do check.

Many of the Indian menus I've seen list that their curries are gluten-free and if they don't, still check and let them know you're celiac when ordering. Obviously, avoid the naan, entrees like samosa, and anything deep fried. Some Indian desserts might contain gluten in the form of suji, a kind of semolina used to make sweet puddings, but other than that, Indian is a pretty safe take-out.

- **Mexican**

Mexican is predominantly composed of spices, vegetables, cheese, avocado, salsa, rice meat, beans, and corn tortillas. There is a local Mexican takeaway store that I go to in Australia called Guzman-Y-Gomez. They are also throughout Australia, Singapore, and Japan. I also eat at Chipotle in the United States, and for both these restaurants, I can eat pretty much everything on the menu except for their tortillas. Other than that, I can eat the burrito bowls, nachos, tacos, salads, and chips. All their fillings are 100% gluten-free.

- **Thai**

When it comes to Thai food, it really is a gamble. There are a number of Thai take-out places around me that offer gluten-free. However, they aren't really celiac friendly. They may swap the sauces for gluten-free versions; however, their ladles and woks can be easily cross contaminated. Have you seen a highly used wok before? It has that black stained and ingrained sauce residue on it. Standard coconut milk curries are usually ok; however, a stir fry is where you can run into trouble.

Beware: sometimes Thai dishes like fried rice or Pad Thai may use eggs from a carton in which case there could be wheat in the mixture.

I've had a situation where I was ordering Thai from a local restaurant. They had always been quite good at guaranteeing the food is gluten-free. However, one day upon ordering, it sounded like a new voice on the phone. She spoke broken English and I stressed as best as I could for the meal to be celiac safe. When I arrived to collect it, I peered in the kitchen and I didn't recognize the chef. I began having massive doubts, so I spoke to the waitress in person and went through the drill with her. She assured me it was gluten-free and that it would be all fine.

Within 20 minutes of eating at home, not only was I having a gluten reaction, I was having an allergic reaction where the back of my tongue and throat swelled nearly shut. My eyes started watering and my ears were so itchy I wanted to stick a screwdriver through them and into my head. I don't have any other food allergies so I'm assuming this may have been from a cleaning chemical. When eating Thai, I now make sure I get the same chef every time.

- **Chinese**

Now, this is a whole different story. Chinese menus are filled with dishes containing gluten, like honey chicken or sweet and sour pork. Dishes featuring sauces may also be thickened with flour. The safest option is to avoid altogether or order something simple and safe like egg drop soup, steamed vegetables, or a seafood/meat rice noodle-based dish without any sauce. This is where your little sachet of emergency sauce in your handbag can come in handy. In all honesty, I haven't eaten at a Chinese restaurant since I was diagnosed, as there really aren't any around that I can trust, so I'm not the greatest authority on safely eating gluten-free Chinese food.

Some fast food establishments are getting better at catering to gluten-free, especially in the United States.

Fast Food Establishments

Fast food establishments are fast, but it doesn't make them healthy. Do you think the meat patty you're getting is actually good quality and nutritious? Do you think the gas ripened factory tomatoes are giving you any benefit? Let's face it, fast food is junk food, no matter how you want to justify it, but we've all been known to crack under pressure and some days, you just want to say, 'Screw it, I'm having a burger and chips.' If that's the case, here are how 3 fast food joints handle food allergies.

- **In-and-Out Burger**

This would have to be one of my favorite places to eat a burger when I crack under pressure.

I was running through the Linq Promenade in Las Vegas and needed a quick bite to eat and thought I'd try In-and-Out. I was quite skeptical at first, but I Googled some info, and sure enough, all the patties and fries were gluten-free. The only thing that wasn't GF was the bun.

The forum said to ask for *'lettuce wrapped'* and mention an allergy (even though we all know it's not) and they would prepare it separately and safely. I was so nervous when making my order that I stuttered a little with embarrassment. However, the lady behind the counter took my order like a pro and with such ease that I relaxed. I soon realized that, unlike in Australia, food intolerances, allergies, and diseases are much more common in the US (obviously due to population) so I really got the feeling they had dealt with this a thousand times and had it all under control.

Turns out they have an *allergy button* you can activate, which means they take further precautions. The chain prides itself on allergy sensitivity; however, still be mindful and check each time.

- **Chick-fil-A**

This popular chicken house has a huge range of gluten-free options that use dedicated fryers. They have hash browns, grilled chicken nuggets, waffle fries, grilled salads, and most recently, added a gluten-free bun, so now you can have an actual chicken burger. A fair amount of their sauces and dressings are gluten-free also.

- **McDonald's**

McDonald's just makes it on the list by a bee's dick. (Aussie humor: a bee's dick is so small that we use it as slang measurement for the insignificance of something).

Not having an In-And-Out Burger chain in Australia to rely on, the next best is McDonald's. You can order their meals bunless (excluding the fries) and hope for the best. Cross contamination is still a risk, so you need to rely on the training of the staff. Once, I was traveling through the countryside and ran out of my emergency food, so I opted to try a McDonald's burger without the bun. I stressed to the boy behind the counter about my celiac and hoped that it sunk in. When I collected my meal, it was one piece of thin patty, a slice of cheese, one half-slice of tomato, and a sprinkle of shredded lettuce. What the…? Shredded lettuce! I was so hungry, I was going to need four of these meals to fill me up. Needless to say, there was no discount on the charge of $8.00 just for that. I think I'd rather starve next time. Overall, I was never really a fan of McDonald's before I was diagnosed and have only tried it once since. It's not my thing and I'd rather eat an apple from a Petrol Station than attempt it again.

Hard Note: Some people may not agree with me on this one, but if you're stuck somewhere and can't find anything that's gluten-free anywhere, then STARVE!

Do not crack under any circumstances. Yes, you might get FANGRY, but you won't die. Drink plenty of fluid instead. Your body can handle a little fasting for a few hours or even a day, but if you crack under the pressure and eat something with gluten, you are putting yourself in harm's way. While panicking constantly about food in your own home can be an overly stressful way to live, being overly cautious when it comes to eating out is a worthwhile approach given the greater risk.

What's the rule? When in doubt, leave it out!

Beware. Just because the label says it's gluten-free doesn't mean it's always gluten-free. Accidents happen and products get recalled. There have been several high-profile cases of lethal anaphylaxis attributed to some big companies. Pret á Manger was in the headlines in October 2018 when a 15-year-old girl died on a plane from her sesame allergy after eating a sandwich. Another person died from a milk allergy after eating a vegan flatbread when milk was not disclosed. If you are doubtful of a dish or a response from waitstaff, then leave it out.

Chapter 19

Yes,
You Can Still Travel Overseas

*D*on't panic. This is just like local traveling, only you're a lot further away. Eeek!

Your first overseas trip might feel a little daunting.

- Perhaps you're worried about the language barrier?

- Perhaps you're traveling to a country that is heavily cultured around bread, like Turkey for example, and concerned about what to eat?

- What happens if you get glutened?

- You might see so much food that you cannot eat and be emotionally pissed off? *(For me, this feeling never goes away.)*

These are the types of thoughts that went through my head when I considered my first overseas trip. After some practice with a few different countries and learning from others, I managed to develop an action plan and I adapt it to suit the country to which I'm traveling.

If I'm traveling to a native English-speaking country, it's a breeze. But if it's a vastly different culture, it takes a little more preparation to ensure a relatively smooth trip.

Hotels and accommodations

Book a room with the amenities you want and be prepared to pay the money for it. Don't be a stingy penny pincher and pester the hotel staff for ridiculous items like a microwave to be sent to your room, along with a kettle and coffee maker, when you're only prepared to spend $100 per night. Just because you have a disease, does not make you entitled.

When spending more than a few days in any location, choosing a room with a small kitchenette can be handy for the obvious reasons. Having a mini bar should definitely be a requirement as you can shove fresh fruit, juices, and snacks in easily enough around the little booze bottles. I find this is helpful for a quick breakfast for a morning on-the-go or when I'm darting back to the hotel before venturing out again; I can re-fuel before the next mealtime.

If you're on a budget, perhaps taking the whole family for a holiday, then eating out for every meal can be expensive. Perhaps you need to rely on the hotels' breakfast buffet to save a few dollars. If this is the case, then the selection you're faced with at the Motel 5 might present some challenges when you see nothing but bread and cereal.

Tip 1

First off, I would recommend carrying some reusable toaster bags. There is a variety to choose from on Amazon. These are handy in the event that there is gluten-free toast, but no gluten-free toaster. You could use these toaster bags in the communal toaster at breakfast time to be safe or if you've thought one step further and packed your own GF bread.

These are handy not just at the hotel but also during the day at cafés. I went to a cafe once that had a lovely gluten-free ham and cheese sandwich in the front display case window (top shelf, of course). I was delighted, so I ordered it along with a coffee. My delight turned to disappointment when the waiter picked it up with tongs and put it in the flat bed toaster, on top of the existing parchment paper filled with crumbs. I went white at the sight and I didn't have the guts to say anything. Needless to say, my husband ended up with a nice hot toasted sandwich and I only had the coffee. If I'd had toaster bags with me at the time, I could have given the waiter one to use. Lesson learned.

Tip 2

Bring a largish handbag (or man-bag) with a container inside. When the wait staff aren't looking, squirrel away some fruit and hopefully some hard-boiled eggs, if they have them. (You paid for the breakfast, you might as well get your money's worth.) I took my nephew from Australia to Orlando to visit the theme parks for two weeks. It was a mega expensive trip and theme park food not only has a theme park price tag, it can, at times, be hard to navigate for gluten-free options amongst 80,000 people.

Each morning at the hotel's buffet, I would squirrel away fruit and eggs for myself, and fruit and muffins for my nephew. We had an untapped supply of snack food for two weeks while roaming around the theme parks. At first, my husband was annoyed and embarrassed at my thriftiness, but that bit him in the ass when he asked me one day, *"Hey, have you got any of those choc muffins from breakfast in your bag?"*

If you are lucky to live the life of luxury, then you have no worries at all. You would have bought the upgraded package for the all-inclusive buffet breakfast to get you going in the morning, which would have plenty of fresh fruit, omelets, and maybe a gluten-free toaster with gluten-free options. The hotel would have a wonderful *a la carte* restaurant that will cater to your desires with waiters dressed like penguins, and a 24-hour room service menu that can cater to your every whim. Simply, you need not worry!

Tip 3

Google the area before booking your accommodation to see what restaurants are around. If you're staying for more than a few days, try to pick a hotel within walking distance to grocery or convenience stores.

Tip 4

Pack emergency food. In most countries to which I have been able to travel, I've always gotten in with a bag of snack bars and protein powder in my checked luggage. Protein powder has been my easy go-to. Just add water and I have a delicious meal that will keep me full.

International flights

My first learning experience started with the airline. Get used to booking a gluten-free meal. Before I was diagnosed, I had never in my life booked a meal on a flight. I used to think that the people who got their meal first before everyone else were such high-maintenance people. *Oh, I need kosher; oh, I need dairy-free,* I would mutter in a hoity-toity tone in my mind. Boy, did I learn my lesson here, too.

I booked my first flight and selected the gluten-free in-flight meal. *Ok, easy enough so far*. On the flight, sure enough, before everyone else got their meals, my gluten-free meal arrived. *This is perfect,* I thought to myself, as I was on an A380 AirBus with 50 million passengers. I comfortably ate my meal before everyone else, then while everyone was busy with their meals and locked in their seats, I had uninterrupted use of the toilet. I then got back to my seat just in time to grab another wine from the drink cart passing by, settled in for a movie, and laughed at the herds of people fighting their way down the aisles to use the lavatory!

Yay, so, being celiac has a plus side finally, I thought. I can't believe I made fun of people for ordering special meals when, in fact, they had it all worked out.

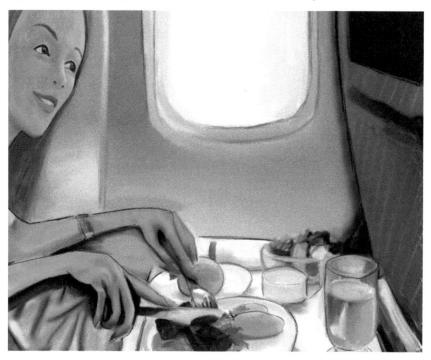

Win number 1

The next time I had to fly to LA, I booked my flight last minute, within 24 hours of departure, and tried to order my gluten-free meal online but I was locked out. So, I called the airline and they responded with, *"We will try to get you a gluten-free meal, but we need 48 hours' notice and cannot guarantee it."* Oh, crap, I thought. *Now what am I going to do? Well, I'll just have to pack a bucket load of snacks to get by, I suppose.*

I boarded the flight, and sure enough, no gluten-free meal for me. But I came up with a devilishly cheeky plan.

I waited till after the dinner service concluded and the staff were able to settle down. I found the oldest male flight attendant and pleaded my case, explaining that I had been working right up until getting on the flight and hadn't had time to arrange anything, all the while batting my eyelashes. I asked if he would happen to have anything he thought might be suitable? He sweetly looked at me and said, *"Honey, I'll go see if there is anything left over from first class. I'm sure there is something there for you to eat."* I brushed his arm with a flirtatious gesture, chuckled a thank you to him, and returned to my seat where my husband was laughing his butt off at me, *thinking* I'd had no luck.

Not long after, the attendant bobbed down beside me as if he was hiding something special that he didn't want the other passengers to see. Sure enough, it was a beautiful ceramic plate with grilled chicken and vegetables, a real linen napkin, silver cutlery, and a glass of champagne. I blew the attendant a kiss and quietly thanked him.

I turned to face my husband with the biggest cheeky grin across my face and saw his jaw drop. To emphasize my win, I made overly loud clinking sounds with my *real* cutlery and sipped obviously from my glass of champagne. He sat back in his seat with a charred, jealous look on his face as he slurped on his plastic sippy-cup of orange juice and pushed away his dried-up muffin. So, being nice to others (and perhaps a little flirty, too) can pay off when you need it.

Win number 2

On another occasion, I was taking a flight to Dubai and again it was last minute and I didn't have time to arrange a meal. I had racked up a few flights that year and was given a lounge access pass for free. Yippee! I got to the lounge extra early and hit the buffet of free food and drinks.

I made up a couple of plates of food from what was there, took it back to my table, and began to perfectly pack my own dinner box into the empty plastic container I had brought with me. I did get a funny look from the waitress as she asked if I would like a beverage, but she was polite enough not to question my behavior; I was in a lounge after all.

Oddly enough, in that moment, I had a strange feeling waft over me. *Oh no, I'm just like my mother,* I thought as I remembered her taking a backpack full of containers to the all-you-can-eat Pizza Hut® night on my birthday when I was a child. I quickly shook the memory out of my head and reconciled to myself: *It's different; I have a* disease.

Win number 3

When traveling back from LA to Australia with my husband, again at the last minute, I couldn't arrange a meal in time. We again went to the airline lounge, but this time I had no containers. My husband urged me to ask the lounge manager if they were able to help out somehow. I put my big girl pants on and looked around for the manager. Sure enough, there was a tall, dark, sexy, chocolate man standing proud in his uniform. Strangely enough, an odd *purr* slipped from my lips that surprised me. *Calm your farm, Jodie, you're spoken for,* I thought. I went up to him, explained my situation, and asked if I could possibly get a container to put some food in. He did one better and said, *"Ma'am do you have any other allergies or food intolerances?"* I replied, *"No,"* and then he said *"I'll have the chef whip you up something special and I'll bring it to you right before you have to leave so it stays hot and fresh. What flight are you on?"*

Damn, is this how the rich people live? Again, having a little luck on my side, I wanted to enjoy this moment as they are very far and few between.

However, now it's time for my luck to run out.

Major loss

On another occasion, I couldn't organize a gluten-free meal in time for a flight and I really didn't have time to go to the shops and pack snacks. I had no lounge passes left and the restaurants in the airport were closed because it was too late. I tried my trick of sweet talking a host to see if I could get a first-class meal, but they were all out. *Oh no!* The host I spoke to said he did have one gluten-free snack box left over that I could have. By now the *fangry* was setting in and I greatly appreciated it.

It was pitch black on the plane, lights out, and everyone was going to sleep. I was starving so much that I opened up whatever was in the packet and shoveled it into my mouth like a senseless teenager.

But as I started crunching I was tasting savory, salty, and dry. *Oh, shit,* I thought, *What is this? It tastes like...pretzels!* My arm shot straight up like a bullet and hit the light button above me, illuminating the entire aisle of the sleeping dead. I stared down at the packet in my hand with crumbs and drool falling out my mouth. It *was* pretzels! I grabbed a napkin and spat out whatever I could in my mouth with an uncouth noise and force as if I'd mistakenly eaten poison. All poise and demeanor went right out the window. I grabbed the small plastic snack box he gave me and there was a banana in it along with this packet of pretzels, but the outside of the container was clearly marked with a gluten-free sticker. *Are you friggin' kidding me?*

I ran to the bathroom to wash my mouth, out and as unpleasant as it may sound, made myself vomit in desperation to try and save myself. After cleaning myself up, I went to the host and said, *"This was not gluten-free!"* He simply apologized and that made me realize that he had no idea of the magnitude of this situation. I went back to my seat and thought, *It's ok, Jodie; you caught it in time, right?...*Wrong.

The shivers started, followed by the sweats, then the stomach cramping set in, and before I could think twice, I ripped the seat belt buckle off in an instant like it was made of tissue paper and ran. I ran down the aisle, jumped like a gazelle over someone's legs, pushed past a drink cart like a bulldozer, and kicked the door into the toilet. My fingers fumbled trying to latch the door shut behind me, all the while squeezing my bum cheeks together with all my might.

The poor passengers seated around the cubicle must have gotten a fright when the plane shook slightly and I emerged again from the remains of another nuclear catastrophe and hoped that no one needed to use the cubicle after me.

There is nothing worse in the history of the world than being stuck on a plane for 14 hours with a crooked gut, farting like a trooper, and running to the bathroom every five minutes like a hungover teenager. My luck had run out and I was taught a very valuable lesson. Check everything first before putting it in my mouth, no matter what the circumstances.

When I got off the flight, I was furious. Not only because of how I felt physically, but I felt a sense of fear over this situation happening to a nut allergy sufferer, and even worse, a small child. I only got sick, and yes, the long-term damage to my villi is bad, but this kind of screw up could seriously hurt someone or even be fatal.

I read an article in the *Standard* newspaper from the UK headlined, *Man served single banana on nine hour-flight after ordering a gluten-free meal,* so I wasn't the only unlucky one.

Not all airlines provide the in-flight service, so pack adequately and always check everything before you eat it.

Win number 4

I'm not one to complain, but I now felt very protective of people with allergies and thought I should write to the airline. I wanted to tell them of this situation so that better training and awareness could be put in place and hopefully keep it from happening to someone with a fatal allergy. So, I did just that. I wrote to the airline about my experience. I wasn't expecting any response, but this is what transpired.

26 Apr 2017, at 6:40 p.m.

Dear Ms. Clapp,

Thank you for your feedback regarding your experience with our airline on 12 March 2017 when you flew from Brisbane to Los Angeles. I am sorry to hear of your ill health and I hope you are feeling better.

We take the safety and wellness of all of our guests very seriously and I confirm we are currently looking into your matter both internally and with our catering provider.

We confirm that we have legal obligations to you, including under the US Department of Transportation's Code of Federal Regulations and you may have a right to pursue action under the non-discrimination provisions of the Code of Federal Regulations.

I will come back to you once we have been able to establish what occurred on board your flight.

Kind regards,

(Name removed)

Then on the 23rd May 2017 I receive this email:

Good afternoon Jodie,

Thank you for your patience regarding your unsatisfactory experience with our airline. I apologize on behalf of the (name removed) group of airlines for the stress and inconvenience caused.

Due to the serious nature of the issues encountered a full investigation was conducted. Based on the information received we believe you were provided the incorrect meal due to the fact it was labeled incorrectly. We have taken this up with our caterers to ensure this does not happen again. Based on the additional checks and balances I'm confident the chances of this happening again are minimal.

I regret that your experience with (name removed) was neither smooth nor met expectations. I therefore wish to offer a $1,000.00 Travel Bank as a gesture of goodwill for future flights. If you would like to proceed with this offer, please contact me directly.

Once again, I apologize unreservedly for the poor experience that you had on this occasion. I do hope that we will have the opportunity to demonstrate our commitment to service excellence on a (name removed) flight in the near future.

Yours sincerely,

(Name removed)

I was completely gob smacked at this response, even though it took a month to hear back. I was so happy to read that better measures were being put in place, not just for me but for others that have more serious conditions. I wasn't expecting any compensation as I believe that I am solely responsible with what goes in my mouth, but hey, I won't turn down a $1,000 flight credit.

Travel cards

If you're in a country that's not English-dominated, you may want to take a travel card with you that details your allergy translated into that country's language. They are small like a credit card and there are various versions you can download off the internet that explain your food restrictions in most languages. celiactravel.com has free cards in 63 languages that you can download, but I do recommend you make a donation if you can.

Here is what the card says:

> *"I have an illness called Celiac Disease and have to follow a strict gluten-free diet. I may therefore become very ill if I eat food containing flours or grains of wheat, rye, barley and oats. Does this food contain flour or grains of wheat, rye, barley or oats? If you are at all uncertain about what the food contains, please tell me. I can eat food containing rice, maize, potatoes, all kinds of vegetables and fruit, eggs, cheese, milk, meat and fish - as long as they are not cooked with wheat flour, batter, breadcrumbs or sauce. Thank you for your help."*

Restaurant cards aren't foolproof, but they do come in handy. There are various other options available on the internet that combine dairy and other intolerances you might have.

Voice translators

Multi-language portable voice translators are amazing. Small enough to fit in the palm of your hand, they can translate your voice in just a second and repeat it in another language. Not only that, but when the person responds in their language, it will convert it back to you in English, giving you a two-way instant speech conversation. The best translators cover over 70 different languages, making them one the best travel investments you can make.

Not only will you be able to communicate your concerns about food easily when dining, you will be able to use it for anything else along your trip like booking transport. Prices for this device cost a bit more than travel cards, ranging from $50 to $200, but so far, the best one I've come across is Mortentr Translator Device Smart Voice on Amazon. However, be mindful. The model you choose will depend on whether or not you need wi-fi or cellular data connected to it.

Gluten-free travel agents

Maybe you're not a savvy intrepid traveler who books everything on your own and you need a little help and guidance. Although the travel agent profession seems to be slowing down, there is now a market for the *free-from* travel agent. There are multiple travel agents on the internet that specialize in gluten-free travel, from cruises to hotels to tours. The best part about an online travel agent is that you don't have to rely on your local operator. You can select a travel specialist from anywhere in the world and easily work with them through the net.

Plan ahead as much as possible

Search for places that other gluten-free travelers recommend. TripAdvisor and gluten-free travel blogs are pretty useful, along with local Facebook groups.

When I am going somewhere new, I'll search for a local gluten-free Facebook group in that area and ask the locals about a good place to eat. Keep a list of cafes, markets, and grocery stores in a notebook or somewhere on your phone accessible off-line, as sometimes you might not have data access.

You can even create your own restaurant guide on Google Maps by pinning various places to the local map. Then print the map so you have the details when not on wi-fi. You can also click on the selected places in Google and then send it to your phone, email, or even save it.

Pinterest is amazing at filtering through information. Just type in gluten-free cities and be surprised at what you find. There are pins like, "The best gluten-free eats in NYC," and "Gluten-free Dublin, Ireland," and even pins like, "Top 10 gluten-free cities around the world." So, when you are looking for a little help, don't forget about Pinterest. It's more than just pretty picture ideas; it's a wealth of articles, news, and resources.

Phone apps are handy

Before going on a trip, especially to somewhere non-English speaking, I like to try and find apps that might be useful.

Find Me Gluten-free is a favorite. I can simply type in *Rome* in the search bar and it gives me a list of places I can eat. If I'm not sure where they are in relation to me, I can just hit the map button and see them all in a map view. The best part is this app is free and by far the best on the market.

Pack your emergency kit

One thing you will need to figure out is your emergency kit. This is a kit with products, vitamins, fluids, and a regimen that will help you overcome accidental gluten exposure. Everyone reacts differently when they are glutened and has their own way of dealing with it. It's worth figuring out what works for you and packing your emergency kit for just-in-case situations.

Aside from my daily vitamin regimen, I pack the following:

1. **E3 Advanced Plus** from Dr. Tom O'Bryan is my savior. It's a formula composed of enzymes, prebiotics, and probiotics designed to break down the gluten proteins. So, if I have a meal and I suspect some contamination, this is the first thing down my throat to give me a hopeful shot at surviving the accidental exposure.

2. **Bi-carb soda/citric acid.** I use a product specifically called Eno. Bi-carb soda has been shown to help move the gut into a more anti-inflammatory state. It helps to relieve the bloated feeling I get and soothes the cramping.

3. **Electrolytes** are handy in case of excessive diarrhea.

4. **Ginger tea** helps with bloating and nausea.

5. **Lemon juice** in water helps to alkalize my stomach and soothe bloating.

6. **Milk thistle tablets** help the liver and kidneys detoxify. When I'm glutened, my blood is obviously getting a dose of toxins, so milk thistle helps the liver and kidneys flush out any toxins, including alcohol.

I get narcoleptic when I'm glutened, and finding transport back to my hotel so I can crash out quickly is really important or I feel like I'll pass out wherever I am. Ensuring you can get back to your hotel safely so you can recover, use the bathroom in privacy, and sleep it off is essential.

Overall, the main things when traveling are to pack your essentials for emergencies, take your travel cards, and do your research before you go.

There will be many things you can no longer eat, which can cause frustration, but food is only one aspect of your trip. With some research on the amazing foods you can have and where to find them, focus on what you can have rather than what you can't, and this extends beyond food. There is still much to be excited about on a trip from people to culture to sites. If you're like me and thrive on those memorable experiences like sitting in a vineyard under the Tuscan sun sipping on rosé while eating pasta, and think that you might never get to do that, guess what? You can, it might just take a little more effort to find.

Chapter 20

My Recipe
for Healing the Body

The unfortunate news is that recovering from celiac disease is not a quick process. Realistically, it can take years.

The following chapters describe the program that I developed for myself. I knew after I picked up that loaf of bread to buy in the supermarket (the one with so many nasty additives) that going gluten-free simply was not going to be enough to fix the damage; it was going to require a multi-angled approach.

To begin with, I needed to cool down the gut inflammation as quickly as possible. The first thing I did was go 100% cold turkey on the gluten and all the other nasties, including corn, soy, and modified starches. If you'll remember from the chapter **The Bonnie & Clyde of Your Guts**, for inflammation to heal, you need to remove the cause. In my case, gluten was one of them, but I also needed to make sure I wasn't going to fuel the fire by eating other inflammatory foods like corn, soy, and modified starches. All were ingredients that make up many gluten-free products.

Around the six to 12-month mark, I started seeing more drastic improvements. My body was stabilizing after the gluten detoxification process, my energy levels were picking up, I was getting used to the idea of this new lifestyle, but mostly, my blood work stabilized. I retained my iron, which meant one thing: my villi were growing back and I was absorbing nutrients from food.

At the 18-month mark, I went and had another biopsy to see the state of my villi. They were there just as they should be—healed and healthy. It seemed that my plan had worked and life became a situation of disease *management* rather than disease *treatment*.

I had set my own expectations of what I wanted to achieve. I guess you could say I mapped out a business plan for my body. *Geek alert!* My goal was to regenerate the villi as fast as humanly possible, reduce the inflammation, and hopefully, heal the leaky gut that I was most likely suffering from too. I wanted my iron to stabilize from the transfusion at the hospital after my diagnosis and didn't want to repeat this process again.

I have no children to worry about, and my husband was happy to eat whatever I ate, so I was free to focus on myself and my plan of action. I know a lot of other people don't have that luxury, so I felt grateful.

So, let's focus on you and what things you might need to consider on your journey:

- Are you already on a particular diet like vegan, vegetarian, pescatarian? Is cutting out gluten going to be a massive change to your current eating regimen?

- Do you have any major allergies, like dairy, to consider and cutting out gluten is another big step?

- Do you live with family, children, or a partner who you need to think of when changing your diet?

- Is everyone in your home able to eat what you eat, or will you need to cook different meals at once?

- Will you have to teach your family members about gluten contamination and storage of gluten containing foods if it remains in the home?

- Will you have to fit more time into your schedule to read books like these and learn more about meal prepping?

These are some of the questions many people will face when they are diagnosed with celiac disease, and unfortunately, there is not a one size fits all rule here.

Quick Tip: If dealing with additional allergies, then I would suggest getting the book series from Loni's Allergy Free to help you on your journey and to join

The GF Hub Facebook community to ask specific questions and gain insight from others in the same situation.

When embarking on your journey, it's important to know and understand your commitment to your condition. Let's face it, people don't usually succeed on diets. Diets are hard; people cheat and fall off the wagon time and time again. Going gluten-free is a commitment to eating a whole new way, not just for months, but for the rest of your life. Adding to that, if you want to be healthy, vibrant, and the person you deserve to be, there is more to learn than just avoiding gluten and it takes much more commitment than a diet switch.

The next few chapters describe the action plan I put in place for myself after diagnosis, which consisted of what food I ate and avoided, my change in exercise and the impact it has on healing the gut, the need for the sun's healing rays, and the addition of supplements to give me the extra boost I needed.

My personal program for success
= Food + Exercise + Sun + Supplements

Disclaimer: *I am not a doctor, nor do I claim to be one. I came up with the following plan that suited me, my body, and my lifestyle.*

Food: the way *I choose* to eat

There is no one size fits all approach to food lifestyles and I don't want to dictate to anyone on how they should eat. However, perhaps if I share the way I choose to eat, there may be snippets of my lifestyle that could be useful? Maybe throughout my experience, there are bits and pieces that might work for you?

Before being diagnosed celiac, I had studied research papers, watched documentaries, and read books on vegan, paleo, all carb, no carb, blood type, keto, raw diets, etc. I tried most of them for long periods of time and not because of a particular belief but rather for fun, research, and maybe to see if one suited me best. My husband used to get so frustrated with me when I would say, *"I'm on a new path with food."* He knew what that meant for him, and that was cutting out the things he usually liked to eat, and listening to me preaching about the latest research article and trying to justify what I was doing. I have to commend the man for his infinite patience with me.

When I think back about this, I realize I was trying to find a place I was comfortable to sit within the many food lifestyles available. I wanted to enjoy the exploration of food but always wanted to eat healthy at the same time. I had seen so much research *and* propaganda that advocated veganism as the right way to eat, then paleo was the right way to eat. Basically, it felt like every diet was claiming to be…the right way to eat.

In trying these different types of food diets, I found they all require significant discipline and each came with their own set of rules. I'm not one who likes rules very much, so I found this challenging.

On the blood type diet, I wasn't supposed to eat tomatoes; yet I love them and they love me, so cutting them out was hard. When I was vegan, I really *craved* eggs. When I was raw, I missed a hearty wholesome hot stew on a cold winter's night. When I was paleo, I missed potatoes.

I did give most of them a good go: I went vegan for nearly a year and for others it was many many months, all in effort to find out what was working for me. In the end, it was a balance of all of them.

Being diagnosed with celiac disease forced me into a new way of eating. Having to cut out gluten meant I really didn't want to be limited too much in any other dietary way, so I found a balanced approach that works for me.

Below are the main elements that make up my diet, and how and what I eat within them.

Meat to vegetable ratio

80/20—I eat 80% plant-based and 20% meat. This simply comes naturally to me and I don't have to think about it, so I just roll with it.

Processed foods

I eat very little processed food or packaged meals, the exception being some brown rice crackers and gluten-free pasta. I do like condiments and I have some cured meats every now and again, but I try to find them nitrate-free. I rarely eat packet processed except for cheat days. Cheat days for me are a Saturday. It's a great way to enjoy a splurge on the weekend after a hard week working and training. I allocate the afternoon for letting loose and enjoying gluten-free burgers and chips, popcorn, ice cream, chocolate, crackers and dips, etc. Essentially, it's my processed food day. Throughout the week, I find it easy not to eat processed foods because I make my own sourdough bread and protein balls, and my meals usually combine salad and veggies. Even on my cheat days, if I'm not eating popcorn and ice cream, I'm eating my own version of crumbed chicken nuggets, or arancini balls. I have a big batch of them in the freezer; they are made with fresh and healthy ingredients and are easy to pull out and air-fry or shallow fry up for what seems like a naughty snack.

Milk / dairy

I choose not to drink cow's milk when possible. I use rice almond milk in my potato mash, coffees, granola, smoothies, etc. I find cow's milk is quite heavy on my gut. I don't like the taste of it anymore, but I also choose not to drink milk for many other reasons. It's not something I find very nutritious. Milk also can cause inflammation, and can rob your bones of calcium. There are other alternatives to cow's milk like almond, coconut, rice milk, etc. You should know by now after reading the soy chapter that soy milk is probably not the best option.

As a teenager, I was told somewhere along the way to have a big drink of whole milk to line the stomach before a heavy drinking night out with friends. Since alcohol is absorbed through the stomach and milk creates an overabundance of mucus production to block absorption, I guess there was some truth to this age-old wives' tale. Since getting older and wiser, I have figured out a few better alternatives.

Cheese also creates mucus production inflammation. But I love it way too much to give it up. I rarely eat supermarket cheese and try to limit myself to once a week. The aged brie I buy is organic from a French fromager at my local farmers market. You know, the real stinky kind that smells like old socks when you unwrap it? It's also fermented and full of bacteria. I know that's not an excuse to eat cheese, but at least it's a better choice over the supermarket products that are mass produced with little nutritional benefit. I'm willing to make a parlay with my body so I can eat a little cheese and still enjoy life.

I've swapped out cow's milk yogurt and replaced it with an amazing coconut version instead. It's lighter on my stomach, full of healthy fats, and very low in sugar.

So, aside from some cheese every now and again, I don't really have much dairy in my diet anymore. One might automatically think, *But what do I do for calcium*? First, there are many other alternatives for calcium like seeds, oily fish, beans, lentils, almonds, leafy greens, rhubarb, figs, etc. I have been off cow's milk for close to 10 years and eat very minimal dairy; not one blood test in that time has ever shown low calcium levels.

Fish

I try to eat wild caught fish when possible. I'm lucky enough to live by the sea where we have trawlers coming in most days with fresh wild caught fish, so I can buy direct. Farmed fish sold in a supermarket as *'freshly caught'* is not as healthy. Thousands of fish cramped into small pens, sometimes not even in the ocean, fed grains and antibiotics…it doesn't sound very healthy, does it? The unfortunate thing, is that in Australia there is a lot of farmed fish imported from Asian countries where perhaps the farming practice standards differ. When I buy fresh caught fish, I try to be mindful of sustainability. Whilst farming practices are sustainable to the earth, sometimes the quality of the fish is not sustainable to our bodies. I purchase my fresh wild caught fish from reputable fisherman who trawl within the sustainable guidelines allowed by our government. The only time I'll eat farmed fish is when I buy salmon. Salmon in Australia is all farmed. It's still not ideal, but I've done my research and have selected the cleanest *brand* I can find. Note how I say *brand*. Yep, Australian salmon is branded. The only place I can find wild caught salmon is in the freezer section of the health food store. It has traveled all the way from Alaska and costs over $100 per kilogram ($50 per pound) compared to $28 per kilo for farmed. When I'm in the USA, I can't wait to buy some wild caught Alaskan salmon from Whole Foods™. You can really see and taste the difference.

Red meat

I always try to eat organic meat when I can afford it; otherwise, it's 100% grass-fed instead. Diligence is needed when selecting grass fed meat as they can usually be *finished* on grain but still promoted and sold as grass-fed. The best way to tell is to first look for the label stating it's grass fed, then ask the butcher if it is 100% grass fed or finished on grain.

I was chatting to a butcher in Tasmania, Australia (home of some of the cleanest meat in Australia) and the owner said that she sources only 100% grass fed meat as some of her celiac clients react to grain fed meat. So, she won't stock it anymore. From my studies and research, I haven't found any conclusive evidence to say that grain fed meat produces an auto-immune response in celiacs that destroys the villi but I do believe, however, that people can react to very poor quality meat with an inflammatory response.

Either way, I know that consuming grain fed is nowhere near as healthy as natural grass-fed meat. When you think about it, it's quite simple. Cows are designed to eat GRASS, not grains and corn. However, some restaurants and butchers advocate grain fed meat as they feel it creates a better flavor. This may be true, but I personally think grass fed meat is much tastier. It's also more humane.

Apparently, it's cheaper to put 100 cows in a small pen close to a slaughterhouse and feed them cheap grain than it is to maintain lush pastures for them to roam in some distant land. Some production facilities will actually put their livestock on a 100-day fattening program right before they are shipped off to slaughter. This means they weigh more and earn more per kilo. But the quality of the poor little moo cow is not so good. The way they are raised is not only inhumane, but it can also lead to diseased cows. I do not support this one little bit. I know they are animals for food, but they deserve to be looked after and treated humanely till the very end.

Chicken and eggs

Chickens can be treated like cows: locked in cages, and fed antibiotics, hormones, and grain. The poor little things are grown in 30 days for slaughter, compared to the natural 90 days. Some can't even stand or carry their own body weight.

At the supermarket, I have a choice of factory-farmed chickens at $10AUS per/kg, or free-range at $16AUS per/kg or organic at $25AUS per/kg.[72] Personally, I buy free-range because it's what I can afford. I would buy organic in a heartbeat if I was making tons of money, but that's not the case. I like to spend more on good quality meat and eat it less, than spend less money on poor quality meat and eat it more. So, I buy my chicken free range like I buy my grass-fed red meat and for the same reasons.

Have you ever seen yellow chicken meat before? In my supermarket, they sell yellow-colored fresh whole chickens. Plastered right across the front of the packet is '*corn-fed.*' Yuck. That's why they are yellow. But apparently there is a market

---

[72] Approximately $7, $11 and $17USD, respectively

for taste over health. Again, chickens were not designed to eat corn or grain, which is exceptionally unhealthy for the bird and again produces poor nutritional meat; they were designed to eat grubs.

As far as eggs go, I'm still confused as to which one came first: the chicken or the egg. *(Joke!)*

I buy free-range eggs from a local supplier where they only have 1,500 hens per hectare.[73] Free-range in Australia can legally mean anywhere from 1,500 hens per hectare to 10,000. Guess which is the better pick? To find this out, check   the carton label, which will sometimes list how many hens per hectare. If you can't find it there, Google the company to see their policy.

The eggs I buy are so delicious, with lovely yellow yolks, not yolks that are bright orange. From speaking with some chicken farmers, the more yellow the yolk, the more grass fed it is. The more orange the yolk is, the more grain fed. In my free-range carton, each eggshell ranges in color, shape, size, and texture. It does cost me an extra $3.00 AUS per dozen, coming in at $9 AUS/dozen, compared to $6 AUS/dozen,[74] but it's well worth it.

Vegetables

Ah, the humble vegetable. I don't think there is a vegetable out there I don't like. When I was growing up, I hated Brussel sprouts, mushrooms, and olives, but oddly enough, love them now. My taste buds have changed so much that the idea of being restricted with gluten taught me to love food I didn't love before. I eat vegetables at least every day in some form and thrive on using rainbow colors in my food. Sometimes when I've *fallen off the food wagon* and have been eating too much take-out or party food for a few days during holiday times, I find myself craving vegetables and will make up a massive vegetable bake, stir fry, kettle of soup, etc. and go vegan for a week. It's not hard to enjoy steamed veggies, baked veggies, stir fry veggies, stuffed veggies, and the list goes on. I can feel the difference when I feed my little gut microbes a dose of veggies over a burger.

Fruit

Fruit is quite a seasonal food for me. I find I eat way more fruit in summer than in winter. In summer, it's in the form of acai bowls and fruit salads for breakfast,

---

[73] Approximately 2.5 acres
[74] Approximately $2, $6, and $4 USD, respectively

and in winter, it might be stewed apples and granola. I don't have much of a sweet tooth so my preference is for bananas, pears, and mangoes mostly, but again, I try to invoke the rainbow principle. The more colors, the better nutritional coverage. I always try to buy in-season produce that's local. Grapes and lychees, for example, are summer fruits, so eating an imported variety in winter doesn't seem to make sense to me. I'm not sure if imported fruit is as nutritional as your local produce. It is grown and harvested under different practices, possibly sprayed with chemicals for shipping to retain freshness, and maybe by now weeks have passed and the nutritional content has diminished somewhat. Fruit that's sold out of season may also be a GMO fruit that has undergone changes to make it grow year-round.

Salad

My gosh, I can never have enough salad. I pretty much eat salad every day for lunch; it is a staple in my diet. It's clean, lean, and makes me feel like a well-oiled machine. I love experimenting with salads in so many ways, much to the boredom of my husband. However, not all salad items are created equal. Salad items can be quite delicate and thus highly susceptible to pesticide residue. Most disappointing is King Kale, which has now made its way onto the dirty dozen list from the Environmental Working Group (EWG) group.

In 2020 more than 92 samples of kale had two or more pesticide residues, and a single sample could contain up to 18 different residues. And that's after washing! According to the EWG group, the most frequently detected chemical was Dacthal (DCPA), which has been classified as possibly cancer-causing by the Environmental Protection Agency (EPA) since 1995 and has been banned for use in Europe since 2009.

The dirty dozen list is a list of produce (vegetables, fruit, salad) that contain the most pesticide residues after preparing, so it's best to buy these organic. View the latest dirty dozen list on my website thegfhub.com

Drinks

Because I don't have much of a sweet tooth, I don't drink much more than water. Water, to me, is the essence of life and I don't know how other people (my mother included) struggle to drink it. I know many people don't like the taste of water and therefore put additives in it like cordial. Typically, cordial is exceptionally high in sugar or High Fructose Corn Syrup and has unhealthy color additives.

I've never really liked fizzy drinks like soda pop and I'm very selective on pre-made juices. They need to be cold pressed, 100% natural, with nothing added. I usually carry a stainless-steel bottle of water in my hand-bag. If I don't, I'll buy water before juice or anything else. I don't mean to sound full of myself with this; I simply like the basics.

I put fresh lemon juice in my water or soda water, which I find keeps my stomach feeling settled. I drink Kombucha or add a concentrated form of fermented juice full of probiotics to my water. And I love herbal teas, especially in winter when it's cold.

Other than that, I try to drink two liters of water every day. Half the time, I'm like every other person out there in this world and don't hit my target due to one excuse or another.

My way of trying to get down 2 liters a day is simple. I have a 1 liter stainless steel can that I fill each morning and my rule is to have it finished by lunch. Then I do the same from lunch till dinner. I usually will only sip water sparingly after dinner as there is nothing worse than having to pee a lot during the night when you're trying to sleep.

I love my coffee and I am not giving it up, no matter what anyone says. I have one mega strong coffee in the morning with rice milk and that's it. It wakes up my brain, keeps me sane, and feeds my addiction.

Alcohol

Oh Alcohol, my faithful little friend. You're with me though my good times and my bad times. You never argue with me and have always been the life of the party.

In all seriousness, though, yes, it causes inflammation. Yes, wine is full of sugar. Yes, it's bad for you in large quantities, but c'mon, surely I can have one naughty vice?

I'm pretty good with everything else yet still want to live life, have fun, and be social, so I will happily enjoy a glass of wine or two with dinner. I pretty much only drink European wine as I don't get as much of a headache or dry feeling like I do from Australian wine. I'm no wine expert, but I would put it down to perhaps less usage of sulfites or better soil. I'm not a big spirit drinker at home and only have them on special occasions with friends. I opt for a nice vodka distilled from rice, guaranteeing it's gluten-free. Thank goodness I found a gluten-free beer that I can enjoy after getting sweaty and dirty mowing the lawn, but this, too, is on the odd occasion. I used to drink way more beer before I was diagnosed, however, options are limited in Australia.

My rule is: booze in moderation and no more than once or twice a week.

Food combinations

One of the things I have noticed when I eat meat is that, if I have some fruit or coconut yogurt for dessert afterward, I get a very upset stomach. It feels like the sugar is fermenting with the meat in my gut and it doesn't really work well at all. So, being the geek that I am, I wanted to learn more about combining foods. However, when reading up about the best food combination practices, I wasn't liking the rules, especially when they said not to combine protein and starch. Screw that! I love, love, love steak and potatoes, and I certainly don't feel sick when eating the two. So, as far as food combinations go, I only have one rule and that is I don't mix fruit or sugary desserts with meals that contain meat.

Mealtimes

Everyone and every diet has a different version of the best practices for meal times.

There is the age-old three-square-meals-a-day rule.

There is the grazing rule of five small meals.

There is the fasting rule of skipping breakfast, and many more options.

For me, I follow all three styles at different times. Some days, I'll have three square meals. Other days, I get hungry sooner rather than later, so I'll graze more. Other days, I know I've over-indulged so I might have a fasting day. I don't have a set way or time of eating; I just eat when I'm hungry. Sometimes, it might be 5 p.m. at night for an early dinner; some days, I don't want dinner at all.

Again, this really just comes down to working with my body. No matter which way I eat, as long as the food is healthy and I'm exercising, I get results. I think fasting can be very essential and important. I have studied the effects it has and it's a very primal way of eating. Think back to hunter-gather days. Do you think the Neanderthals could rock up at McDonald's and order a cheese burger 24/7? Sometimes, a day or even several days may pass until they could catch their next meal. The only thing with fasting for me is I turn into a crabby bitch when I don't get to eat and usually feel a bit weird. But then, for some reason, the following day, I feel the best I've felt in a long time. So, while I know the amazing benefits of it, it's something I only do when I feel I need it rather than making it a part of my weekly lifestyle. Again, each to their own and adopting a 5:2 system (5 days on, 2 days off), or the 16-hour system (only eat within a 16-hour window) might be better for you.

Overall:

When I was vegan, I missed meat.

When I was paleo, I was eating too much meat.

When I was raw, I missed a hot vegetable stew in winter.

When I was doing the carb diet, I was cranky.

When I was doing the blood type diet, I was just weirded out that a tomato was bad for me and I rejected the idea.

When I tried keto, I gave up early because I wasn't allowed wine and stomaching a cup of butter in my morning coffee made me gag.

So, now I have stopped stressing myself out with all of that and just follow *my* guidelines on food that works for *me*. And that's just what they are, *my* guidelines. I am not the picture of perfect health. I am not a Jillian Michaels. I splurge on naughty food and I drink. I have my ups and downs in life and sometimes I don't exercise as much as I should, but I try to do my best, most of the time, to stay on track.

So, what about you? Do you have any thoughts and ideas on how you want to change the way you eat? Do you want to start formulating your own guidelines?

Don't let the idea of learning about food overwhelm you. You don't have to follow a seven-day, 14-day or 21-day program to feel better but rather perhaps just start looking at food in a different way. Prepare meals more from scratch rather than buying a ready-made meal. Make a goal to eat less processed foods. Perhaps change the amount of meat you eat to better quality. Start learning to read the backs of labels of ingredients and perhaps swap some food items for a healthier version with less sugar or fewer additives, for example. Once you start to make better choices with food, it's amazing how the body tells you what it *doesn't* like when you eat something wrong later.

A little story of discovery and learning: I have a close friend of mine who is a shining example of health. She was an endurance horse racer in Dubai and now runs her own acupuncture clinic in Australia. She eats exceptionally healthy, way better than me, and hardly drinks. She has been diagnosed celiac for nearly 10 years, but over the past few years she has been struggling with her health, her energy, and reporting excessive bloating, tiredness, and so on. No matter what approach she took, she couldn't find the cause. After multiple scans and physicians appointments she has only now discovered that soy, and in particular soy lecithin, seems to be the culprit.

As we know, soy is in so many products and especially processed foods. She didn't consume processed foods often, but sometimes, the gluten-free bread she ate had soy in it or the crackers she would have also contained soy. It only took a small dose of soy every few days to a week to keep her feeling unwell during that time. Since discovering this and removing what little she ingested from her diet, she has already shown much improvement.

This is just an example of how inflammation works, and that even some of the healthiest of us still have struggles and are still learning along the way. The more we can share stories like these, the more we can all learn from each other.

Exercise: it's more than shedding dimples from your butt

Exercise is such an important factor in health, not only for the obvious appearance reasons, but it's also good for the gut. Regular exercise has been shown to help boost beneficial bacteria[75] in the gut and promote an anti-inflammatory environment.[76] There appears to be a strong link between obesity and an unbalanced gut,[77] and this is something we don't seem to hear much about.

Aside from eating better foods to balance out the gut, exercise plays an important role. When you exercise, fat-blasting microbes start to multiply and call your gut home. These little fat-blasting critters gobble up your carbohydrates

---

[75] Monda V., Villano, I., Messina, A., et al. (2017). "Exercise Modifies the Gut Microbiota with Positive Health Effects." *Oxid Med Cell Longev,2017*:3831972. doi:10.1155/2017/3831972
[76] Beavers, K.M., Brinkley, T.E, and Nicklas, B.J. (2010). "Effect of exercise training on chronic inflammation." *Clin Chim Acta., 411*(11-12):785–793. doi:10.1016/j.cca.2010.02.069
[77] Davis, C.D. (2016). "The Gut Microbiome and Its Role in Obesity." *Nutr Today, 51*(4):167–174. doi:10.1097/NT.0000000000000167

(starches) and rule over your fat-storing nasty microbes. The more beneficial fat-blasting microbes you have, the less dimples you will have on that butt of yours and the better your gut is going to feel.

Carrying excess weight around your midsection can have a not-so-good effect on your gut. Extra weight can put pressure on your stomach, and if you're wearing tight pants to accommodate the extra weight, it can be even worse. Your poor stomach can be squashed, pushing food back up and into your esophagus along with the stomach acid, causing heartburn.

Overall, regular exercise can:

- Make you feel happier by releasing that wonderful drug serotonin, giving you the *'I can conquer the world today'* feeling.

- Increase your bone mineral density to fight against age and osteoporosis. This is a key point for sufferers of celiac disease to focus on if they have low density.

- Reduce your risk of chronic disease by reducing inflammation.

- Increase your viral fighting immune system.

- Keep your brain sharp as a tack for focus.

- Keep your memory alive so you can recall happy times and fight dementia.

- Help you sleep better at night so you're not such a grump during the day.

- Boost your energy levels so you're more productive.

- Elevate your sex drive. Who doesn't love sex?

- Clear your skin from the pizza and beer you had the night before.

- Detoxify your blood.

I could write a hundred reasons why exercise is so important, but for the most part, let's think about how good it is for your gut, which is the main issue we are dealing with here.

Once upon a time, I used to be crazy about fitness. When I was 18, I completed a Diploma of Exercise Science and I went into personal training for a couple of years. However, life changed for me in that time and I was thrust into the corporate world and gave up being a PT.

While leading a sedentary corporate job life, I always tried to maintain some physical fitness, but I'll admit I'm certainly no saint or athlete when it comes to exercise. I'd be lying if I didn't say that I had my ups-and-downs and ons-and-offs. One month, I'm fighting fit and the next, I'm sitting in front of the computer for 12 hours a day, feeling like crap, eating one too many gluten-free pizzas and complaining about how bad I feel.

I'll admit I've always struggled with consistency. My life and my work are nothing but inconsistent. Aside from work being my biggest issue, I'm also at the mercy of catching a cold or flu like everyone else. I'm also IGA-deficient, meaning when I get sick with the cold or flu, I'll have it for a really, really long time.

Excuses, I know!

It would be nice to make out I'm a body-perfect, fit woman, and or tell you I'm Instagram famous for my abs. But I'm not. I like exercise and thrive when I'm in a routine. When something breaks that routine, it's hard to get it back again. The first few weeks of having to haul my butt out of the seat and put my running shoes on really sucks. I would sometimes make up any excuse to myself to not exercise. *"Oh, I have a lot to do today, so I don't have time"* or *"I don't feel so well, I'll start tomorrow."* But once I've gotten over the hurdle of the first few weeks, I crave it. I can't get enough of it. I want more. I see results. I feel better and it's working for me.

But, in an effort to heal my gluten-ravaged body, I really had to change my workout routine from what was a more vigorous CrossFit™-type training, to more jogging, cycling, paddle boarding, body weight, yoga, and calmer-style exercise routines. Turns out, the way you exercise can have an effect on your stress-hormones and also your gut microbes.

I'll admit, I loved CrossFit™. *"Look at me, I can climb a rope right up to the top of the roof and flip giant tractor tires over and over down a car park. Hooraahhh!"* I'd shout as I beat my hands on my chest like Tarzan. Ok, so I really didn't beat my hands on my chest, but I did do all those other things and it was fun and I was strong.

That type of training can be good in *some* cases for *some* people. However, I learned it was not for me while I had a raging gut fire that needed to put out. I learned that those types of short, fast, and heavy weighted movements in the CrossFit™ classes can cause an increase in acid production and slow down the digestion process. Your body needs to eliminate waste and has a process it needs to follow. When you do that kind of training, you put your body in a constant state of needing to eliminate the waste of lactic acid. When this occurs, other parts of the waste removal system in your body have to switch off, or slow right down. Digestion is one of them. It was simply additional stress on my body that I didn't need. Plus, I was almost at the tipping point of going from fit and toned to muscly and thick if I kept pushing it. So, this was something I needed to put on ice for a while and change my game plan. Once you've got your gut issues under control, resuming this kind of exercise should definitely be something achievable.

Yoga, on the other hand, is especially healing for the body due to its calm stress relief, lengthening, and core focus principles. Other more milder types of exercise that I mentioned above like jogging, cycling, paddling boarding, and swimming can reduce inflammation markers in the body. It was still important for me to get my heart rate up and stay strong, just in a different, more gentle way.

I really delved into other types of training, especially body weight training. Geek alert! I came up with my own body weight training system called 'The 500' and think I'll put it out there to the world in another book soon.

I like to mix up my exercise regimen on a weekly basis and this is what it looks like:

- 5 km jog most mornings with fast bursts and maybe some hill jogs
- mountain bike ride once a week or fortnight
- yoga 1 to 2 times a week in the evening
- body weight training regimen 3 to 4 times a week
- stand up paddle boarding (summer only; I'm a wuss in winter and don't like the cold water)
- mountain hiking (I try to fit in every 2 or 3 weeks)
- gym 3 to 4 times a week

It may look like a lot, but it's not really. These items only make up about an hour each and I pick and choose regularly what to do that day depending on work and weather. On most days, I pair a morning run with some body weight exercise or the gym. Some days, I'll do yoga at night. The weekends are reserved for the hiking and biking.

Are there days where I don't? Yes, and that's ok, as long as I'm exercising more days out of the week than not. Then I'm happy.

Everyone is different in their routine and the above is simply mine.

My only suggestion is that, whatever form of exercise you choose to do, make it something that you can do daily or weekly, continuously and ongoing. If you want to take up walking, then keep walking and make it a part of your lifestyle. If you want to take up boxing, then the same thing applies. But whatever you choose to do, do it well and do it often.

If you want or need to lose weight, then look at it as a long-term plan. Guess what will happen if you try and go to the gym seven days a week, and eat lettuce and protein shakes for a month? You *will* lose weight BUT you will also gain it all back and maybe more when you stop, as you won't be able to continue that lifestyle forever. You will probably get sick and stressed out, and once the weight is back, you'll feel like it never worked in the first place and was a big waste of time, so what's the point? Take a breath...

If you change your lifestyle to integrate achievable daily and weekly exercises, combined with an improvement on your food intake, then you might find you get gradual yet long lasting results. Don't forget, it's not all about the way you look but how you feel about yourself and your lifestyle.

I don't have the perfect body. I'm not as lean as a fitness model, but I'm also not overweight either and do try to maintain a body shape and fitness level that I'm happy with. I'm just me. I have a balanced size, I'm proud of my long legs and flat stomach. I work for it. I also work my mouth with food indulgences that result in a few dimples on my butt!

I'm not too strict on myself. If I want to have a binge night on cheese and wine and wake up with a hangover where I can't train, I will. Without regret. And I accept a headache in exchange.

Overall, just changing your diet is not going to be enough to live a long and healthy life. Exercise is absolutely crucial.

Sun: get your daily dose of sunshine

Is the sun friend or foe?

Sun and vitamin D are absolutely essential to human life. The sun can make you feel happy and it's not myth, it's science.

Have you noticed that sometimes when it's stormy or raining that your energy levels are down? You might feel lethargic and want to curl up on the couch and watch a movie. This feeling is not just your imagination. When it's dark outside, you secrete melatonin, which is a hormone that helps control sleep patterns. On the flip side, when it's sunny outside, light enters the eyes and stimulates a part of the brain that influences serotonin secretion and gives you that awesome feel-good feeling.[78]

However, not getting enough of that feel-good sunshine can result in some adverse health effects, with the main one being vitamin D deficiency.

Unfortunately, celiacs—including undiagnosed celiacs—can have an increased risk of vitamin D deficiency, which can lead to osteoporosis. Studies show that vitamin D deficiency occurs in over 60% of diagnosed celiac disease patients.[79] The issue with the ongoing vitamin D deficiency may be from continued malabsorption, lack of sun, and proper dietary intake.

Vitamin D comes from the sun, as I'm sure you know, *and our food.* The only problem is that, with the raging fire in your intestines, there is a chance you're struggling to absorb the vitamin D from the food you eat, hence the most common cause of vitamin D deficiency is malabsorption.

I wouldn't be surprised if you were thinking that you probably don't get enough sun exposure either. I know I certainly don't at times, especially in winter when I leave for work before the sun is up, work inside an office all day, and then arrive home after dark.

---

[78] Lambert, G.W., Reid, C., Kaye, D.M., Jennings, G.L., and Esler, M.D. (2002). "Effect of sunlight and season on serotonin turnover in the brain". Lancet, 360(9348):1840-1842. doi:10.1016/s0140-6736(02)11737-5
[79] Kemppainen, T., Kröger, H., Janatuinen, E., et al. (1999). "Osteoporosis in adult patients with celiac disease". Bone, 24(3):249-255. doi:10.1016/s8756-3282(98)00178-1

After I was diagnosed, I made sure to check my vitamin D levels. The results said I was at the very low end of the normal range. I didn't want to be 'normal.' I wanted to be 'optimal,' so this meant I needed to boost up the D.

Being deficient in vitamin D is just another nail in the coffin when it comes to your health. A vitamin D deficiency can increase your chances of problems like joint pain, osteoporosis, other auto-immune diseases, cancer, heart disease…the list goes on. It makes sense when you think about it really; nearly all life on the surface of the planet requires the sun for survival. Plants, organic matter, bacteria, and us.

If you're deficient in vitamin D and have a raging gut fire going on, supplements may not be the best approach. Chances are, if you're not absorbing D from your food because your villi are worn down, you may not absorb it from supplements either.

Despite contrary opinions, I believe in the old school approach.

Sun bathing.

The most natural and cost-effective solution to boost your vitamin D stores is to get out in the sun and I mean *without* sunscreen. Yes, you heard me right! NO SUNSCREEN. Just let those warm golden rays hit your skin!

Now, before you think of leathery skin, wrinkles, and melanoma cancer, everything needs balance and moderation. That includes sun exposure too. I explain in detail further on how to get this balance without causing you harm.

Sunscreen

First off, let's talk about the elephant in the room. Sunscreen.

How awesome do those fun-in-the-sun-commercials on TV look like for sunscreen? What about the stand at the local chemist selling sunscreen with the bright beach umbrellas and tasseled towels on display? My generation has been taught to slather on sunscreen to block the sun from hitting our skin to protect us from skin cancer, however, there is another edge to the sword. Typical sunscreen has a concoction of toxic ingredients like these: butyl methoxydibenzoylmethane, methylbenzylidene camphor, octocrylene, aluminum, and oxybenzone.

That's a complete mouthful to try and say! These ingredients share a common value. They are toxic. Between these ingredients, they mimic estrogen, cause cell damage, block vitamin D, promote the growth of cancer cells, cause inflammation, neurotoxicity and…and…and…

A study by Margaret Schlulmpf, PD Dr.sc. nat. ETH in 2010 found that at least one sunscreen chemical was present in 85% of Swiss breast milk samples, indicating that the developing fetus and newborn may be exposed to these chemicals![80]

We weren't designed to avoid the sunlight all together, otherwise we would be at the bottom of the ocean like some archaic squid with no eyes living in blackness. Yet some people avoid the sun like the plague, (and some for good reason, due to particular skin conditions). However, when some people do venture out in the sun, out comes the sunscreen that is slathered from top to toe on every inch of flesh exposed to the sun. So, whilst one might want to protect themselves from the sun, they also may be doing themselves an injustice with the amount of toxic chemicals that are being put on their skin.

The most effective way of protecting your skin is the 'cover up method.' Hat, sunglasses, long sleeve shirt, etc. If you really feel the need to get slathering slop happy then zinc oxide is the best. Just plain old zinc is a natural element found on the periodic table of elements with the symbol Zn. It is also helpful in healing the body, supporting the immune system, is anti-inflammatory, and is an antioxidant.

Zinc oxide is zinc combined with oxygen molecules, heated, then evaporated, which results in a fine white powder. Now the zinc oxide can be added to creams and other products to help protect the body. Zinc oxide lowers skin inflammation conditions like rosacea, improves wound healing, and protects against skin cancer along with many other benefits too long to list.

How do you get vitamin D from the sun?

When the sun's (UVB) rays hit your body, your body secretes a special molecule of cholesterol on your skin. This cholesterol is mixed with the vitamin D from the UVB to create vitamin D3. This is then absorbed into your body and

---

[80] Schlumpf, Margret & Kypke, Karin & Wittassek, Matthias & Angerer, Jürgen & Mascher, Hermann & Mascher, Daniel & Vökt, Cora & Birchler, Monika & Lichtensteiger, Walter. (2010). Exposure paterns of UV filters, fragrances, parabens, phthalates, organochlor pesticides, PBDEs, and PCBs in human milk: Correlation of UV filters with use of cosmetics. Chemosphere. 81. 1171-83. 10.1016/j.chemosphere.2010.09.079.

broken down by various organs, like your liver, to produce the chemicals your body needs to function.

Getting a safe dose of sun

I knew I wasn't getting enough sun, so as part of my healing regimen, I added some naked sunbathing into the mix, much to my husband's delight. Once a week, typically on a weekend, during the hours of 10am and 2pm when my shadow is shorter than me, I sunbathe for 10-15 minutes on each side of my body. It's not long and this gives me just enough to bead a light sweat for my cholesterol to form. Then I'm back inside again. It's best to leave the sweat beads on the skin for as long as possible, so don't wash them off right away. This lets the body do its absorption processes properly. For me, a bit of sunbathing has nothing to do with getting a tan and that's far from my objective. It's simply the way I like to get a dose of sun. As I work inside an office all the time, I like the feeling of warmth all over my body for just a brief moment, even if it's once a week. Sometimes, it's just not practical to get your clothes off in the sun, so simply reading a book, going for a walk, sitting in the park and soaking up some rays in a way that works for you are other approaches. People also have varying types of skin. I have a skin type that does not burn easily, yet my husband has red hair and white skin. His tolerance level is all of five minutes in the sun before he starts to crisp up like KFC™. So, everyone is different and their needs are different.

I don't ever extend my time in the sun longer than that. I don't want to overcook myself and start to accelerate the aging process or cause any harm to my body. Remember, sometimes too much of a good thing, can lead to a bad thing. Now that I'm better informed, my days of lathering up the coconut oil and laying in the sun for hours are long gone.

What about a day at the beach?

For the first 15 mins to half hour, I'll run around without sun protection on, just a bikini. Then, after that, I'll put on some zinc cream and in most cases, a light t-shirt, hat, and sunglasses. If I'm at the beach with family, I've usually packed a large umbrella so I can go swim and play, but then get back in the shade.

Have I been caught out before? Yes! I have been burned to a crisp where I look like a shining red beacon in the night with a glow in the dark butt. On average, I probably get a roasting for my slackness maybe once every couple of years, so that's not too bad especially considering the Australian sun is so strong. The main thing though is to try and limit the amount of times these accidents happen as they can have some long term implications if you are not careful.

In summary, I love my skin and want to take care of it. But getting enough sun to keep me healthy and happy is really important as well and makes up a big part of my healing regimen.

What about Vitamin D from food?

Sometimes, we just don't have sunny days for weeks or are too busy with life's duties to get out in the sun on a weekend off, so why not boost your vitamin D with food? Your villi may be worn down, you may be suffering from malabsorption, but as you heal, this will get better, so why not flood your diet with vitamin D rich foods for when you can and will start to absorb it again?

Salmon, herring, sardines, cod liver oil, canned tuna, eggs, and mushrooms all contain high levels of vitamin D. Here's the interesting part: to help vitamin D assimilate properly, you need calcium. So, why not combine foods rich in vitamin D with foods rich in calcium like leafy greens, beans, lentils, seeds and nuts.

Bottomline: It might be worth getting your vitamin D levels checked out to see if you are deficient and then making an action plan to raise your levels if need be.

Supplements—power up

Quick little disclaimer: I have not been paid to include any of the products or brands listed here. It would be great if I was, as a little extra cash would be nice. So, this is not a skewed or biased view or an 'influenced recommendation.' This is simply my personal supplement regimen I researched to suit my needs. I'm not a doctor, so I can't really say what you should and shouldn't do, but maybe there might be something of interest here for you to look into.

As we've talked about so much in this book, *inflammation* was a key factor I wanted to address, so I researched the best supplements to help:

1) reduce inflammation by creating an antioxidant environment, and

2) cool the inflammation down.

Leaky gut was another major point I needed to address, so I had to find something that could help 'knit' back the tight junctures that were holding my intestinal wall together. I needed to supercharge my bacteria and get them thriving again. Remember, I'd just gone cold turkey on the main food sources they'd been living on for 30 years, so I best feed them something good and get them flourishing again.

Essentially, I made a list of all these elements and more, then spent a lot of time researching the best approach I could find to suit. I talked to specialists, naturopaths, and nutritionists and gained insight from all of them so I could develop the right path for me.

A note on supplements…they can be hit and miss. In my case, I was anemic, so oral iron supplements were of no help to me at all. Instead, I was given an iron IV transfusion.

In the event that the villi are destroyed, there are functional medicine doctors who can administer IV vitamin therapy and this may help. It's more widely practiced in the United States and Europe than in Australia. In Europe, there are even high dose vitamin IV treatments for cancer. In Australia, a few clinics exist, but the practice is hardly recognized. In the United States, you can get tailored treatments for illness, beauty, and even to cure hangovers (this one I know from personal experience).

Imagine how good it would be to have a high dose of vitamin C and antioxidants in your blood before going on that long-awaited holiday overseas to prevent catching a cold or flu. Imagine when your villi are destroyed and you're incapable of absorbing nutrients properly; you could get a vitamin boost up until you're healed.

Ok…I got side tracked….sorry. Back to *oral* supplements.

If our bodies were incapable of absorbing any nutrients at all, we would probably be dead not long after, so it stands to say that some nutrients do get absorbed. Once you cut out gluten completely, immediately your intestines begin to regenerate and with that regeneration is the ability to absorb more nutrients.

Below was my supplements regimen for the first six months after diagnosis. My goals were to sooth the inflammation, reduce the harmful bacteria that was floating around, and repair my gut lining. I also wanted to replenish my system with good bacteria and nutrients.

My little protocol had a system.

Super Boost – Replenish – Repair - Nourish & Tighten - Support.

WEEK 1

Super Boost

"UltraBiotic 500" from BioCeuticals.

I put myself on a seven-day super course of probiotics containing 14 strains of 500 billion bacteria to kick start my gut flora. This treatment wasn't cheap and cost around $80 for the seven sachets for the week.

Probiotics have been shown to help in:

- reducing inflammation

- the production of vitamins from malabsorption

- breaking down toxins

- keeping the bad bacteria under control

- teaching your immune system to distinguish between harmful and non-harmful pathogens thus helping your immune system to stop overreacting to allergies

- boosting your gut's immune protection system.

WEEKS 2 TO 26

Replenish

"UltraBiotic 45" from BioCeuticals.

This was a step down after the super course and consisted of 10 probiotic strains delivering 45 billion beneficial organisms. I thought of these little critters as my daily gut food.

Repair

"CytoPro Repair" from Eagle.

This is a powdered drink to help repair the gut lining and to help 'knit' it back together. This powder supplement is made up of many herbs and nutrients with a high dose of glutamine to aid in the cooling of the intestinal tract. It also repairs the gut wall lining junctures by increasing the thickness of the cells.

Reduce inflammation

Curcumin is one of the main components found in turmeric and is highly anti-inflammatory.

Turmeric, a vegetable root, has been used for centuries in many different forms, from use as a spice in cooking to use as a pigment for dying and coloring. It was also used in ancient Ayurvedic medicine as an antiseptic for cuts and burns and a remedy for gastrointestinal discomfort and respiratory conditions.

It fights against free radical damage and has been known to play a vital role in fighting off disease, preventing cancer growth, and improving brain and skin health among many other benefits.

Nourish and tighten

Collagen to repair the gut lining.

Collagen is derived from bones, cartilage, and tendons. It helps to boost your gastric juices and contains the amino acids proline and glycine which are the building blocks to repair the damaged intestinal lining. Collagen dates back thousands of years. Do you ever remember seeing a movie based around the time of kings and queens, when a knight would ride into town after a long journey and be offered a bowl of broth? Broth is high in collagen.

Collagen is a natural protein found in our bodies but as we age the production is diminished and the evidence is written all over your face with the appearance of lines and wrinkles. Literally, the degradation of collagen is one of the leading causes of saggy skin.

Taking collagen can not only help to tighten your intestinal wall junctures, it can possibly help to tighten and tone your skin. It's one of the oldest traditional foods in history! I've been taking a marine collagen powder drink backed up by collagen in my foods in the form of bone broth, collagen gummies, and stews. You can make your own bone broth, or you can buy an organic one from the health food store. I just love heating these up, chucking in some vegetables, salmon, and Konjac noodles to make a nice Asian-style broth.

Collagen gummies (not the candy gummies) are a nutritious little treat. It's as simple as boiling up some collagen powder in water, adding in some blended fruit like blueberries or strawberries, pouring it into an ice cube tray and putting it in the fridge to set. They come out like little jellies and I usually snack on these throughout the day.

Support

Ki Immune Defence and Energy Formula as an antioxidant.

I take this particular product from Martin and Pleasance™ as it contains 5 grams of Astragalus, 3 grams of Shiitake mushroom, and 2 grams of olive leaf.

Shiitake contains compounds that have the ability to reduce inflammation, bad bacteria, viruses, and contain essential B Vitamins. Astragalus has a powerful anti-fungal protein. It's also anti-inflammatory, boosts the immune system, and has cancer-preventing properties. Olive leaf is a powerful antioxidant and again, also anti-inflammatory. This product is my go-to, especially when I travel. I take these every day for the previous week to boost my immune system.

6 MONTHS TO 12 MONTHS

This is pretty much the same as the first six months, however I swapped out the CytoPro repair and included spirulina. Spirulina is one of the most amazing foods on the planet.

It's a blue-green algae water plant that is now grown in most parts of the world (tropical climates preferable). It contains nearly all the elements of the ultimate whole food: a large amount of protein, vitamins, minerals, salts, carbohydrates, trace elements, and essential fatty acids.

Spirulina is also super rich in Vitamin B12, which is very beneficial as many celiacs can have a B12 deficiency. If all the food on the planet were to die off, there is a high possibility that we could survive on this one plant alone due to its amazing composition. It comes in tablet or powder form, usually in 500mg or 1000mg. I only get mine from a reputable organic supplier. The health practitioner I purchased this from advised me that this product takes under 20 minutes from harvest to being pressed into powder form.

I could go on and on about the benefits of spirulina, but just Google it for yourself. If you're ever going to take a multivitamin, let it be this one.

I also added in a high strength fish oil. Surprisingly enough, quite a few celiac disease symptoms are linked with a deficiency in omega-3 fatty acids. Quite a few of the other auto-immune diseases like heart disease, diabetes, Irritable Bowel Syndrome (IBS), even obesity and cancer can all be related to omega-3 deficiencies.

Fish oil is amazing at reducing inflammation and is widely recommended for those with chronic inflammation (celiacs). It has many other health benefits like reducing LDL (bad cholesterols), treatment of heart disease, weight loss, improved immunity, reducing arthritis, soothing stomach ulcers, fighting acne and cancer. Fish oil is very important for your brain. For your brain to function well, it needs a few key ingredients like water, salt, and fat. Fish oil has been known to help prevent Alzheimer's disease. So, with that long list of benefits, it seemed to be a good all-rounder for me.

My daily routine for 6 to 12 months

- 1 x probiotic
- 4 x 1000mg spirulina tablets
- 1 x curcumin (I like to use ones with black pepper for better absorption)
- 2 x 2000mg high strength fish oil
- Ki Immune Defence and Energy Formula
- collagen gummies

12 MONTHS AND BEYOND

It was at the 18-month mark when I went back to hospital for another intestinal biopsy to see how my avoidance of gluten-containing foods and intake of supplements was working, and this was the result:

> *"The specimen container is labeled 'Small bowel bx.' The specimen consists of three portions of pink tan tissue measuring from 2mm to 5mm in greatest dimension.*
>
> *The sections show fragments of small intestinal mucosa with preserved villous architecture. No parasites or granulomas are identified. There is no evidence of epithelial dysplasia or malignancy."*

Yeehaa! Preserved villous architecture and no epithelial dysplasia is a great result! This is such an improvement to the first biopsy saying "100% atrophy of the villi."

It would appear that I really was on the right track. I now needed to work on a life-long management program. I've developed the following supplement regimen that I alternate depending on seasons, my overall fitness level, and whether or not I've been drinking too much alcohol over the holidays.

I decided on an everyday program that I'd take to maintain my gut and overall health, however, I tended to add in some different herbs, vitamins, and minerals depending on what's going on. For example, when my husband comes back home from working overseas for a couple of months, we eat a lot of cheese, savories, wine, and naughty pastas and pizzas. We practically have 'date night' every night, so after a week of this, I need to get myself back to normal. To do this, I might take some minerals like chromium to help with the cravings and balance my blood sugar spikes. I might take some other herbs like milk-thistle to help detoxify my liver. Usually at this point my skin is terrible again so I'll want to boost it up also. I also travel a lot overseas, so I'll add in some extras a couple of weeks before to boost up my immunity.

You might wonder, *If I eat healthy enough, then do I really need all these supplements?* My answer is this: even if we eat organic, if we can afford it, our food is not as nutritiously full of vitamins and minerals as it once was. Our soils are depleted of nutrients and bacteria that's important for the growth of food.

Remember what I mentioned earlier about the bowl of spinach? I also don't want to 'survive' or be 'normal,' I want to be *'optimal.'*

My 'Every Day Non-Negotiable' Regimen

1. Spirulina

2. Fish Oil

3. Probiotic

4. MSM Powder (Methylsulfonylmethane)

5. Vitamin B Complex

MSM is a naturally-occurring sulfur found in plants, animals, and humans.

It's found in all the cells of our body and mostly concentrated in our muscles, skin, and bones. It's an important constituent of connective tissue and cartilage and necessary for the formation of protein fibers that hold connective tissue together. I take it for the purpose of supporting the health of my digestive tract lining, for its anti-inflammation properties, and to work in helping to maintain my tight-junctures and to help fix and prevent leaky gut syndrome.

Other benefits of MSM include:

- treatment of osteo-arthritis and joint pain

- repair skin problems like rosacea

- reduce allergies

- aid in wound healing

- lower muscle pain and spasms

- restore hair growth through boosting keratin

My 'Want to Make My Skin Shine' Regimen

1. Evening primrose oil

2. Silica

Evening primrose oil contains a high amount of gamma linolenic acid (GLA). GLA is an essential fatty acid found in hemp seed, borage, blackcurrant seed, and the evening primrose plant. It's an omega-6 oil like DHA from fish oil, however,

GLA is most effective in regenerating the skin, treating skin disorders like acne and dermatitis, and retaining moisture. Aside from being super effective for the skin, it can also improve various other conditions like rheumatoid arthritis, breast cancer, hypertension, diabetic neuropathy, menopause, PMS, osteoporosis, and ADHD.

Silica is the third most abundant trace element in the body after iron and zinc. Silica is imperative for building and maintaining collagen. Silica not only helps keep teeth, nails, and hair strong and robust but also is anti-inflammatory and helps with skin conditions. Silica also keeps other minerals in balance like calcium and magnesium and helps to regulate your hormones.

After your mid-twenties, silica diminishes just like collagen so it's a good idea to boost it up. Silica carries more oxygen to the cells, so combined with better hydration retention, the appearance of fine lines starts to diminish, and the skin takes on a more youthful glow. Silica is also great for the gut lining.

My 'I'm Training Very Hard and Need Support' Regimen

1. Branched chain amino acids (BCAA)

2. L-glutamine

3. Hydrolyzed collagen peptide protein

4. Magnesium

There are 20 amino acids that make up the proteins in your body and are broken down into 3 categories.

- Essential Amino Acids: cannot be made by the body so you need to absorb them from food.

- Non-essential Amino Acids is when your body produces them on its own regardless whether you eat it in food or not.

- Conditional Amino Acids: typically are non-essential, but when the body is under trauma or stress these need to kick up a gear and supplementation from food.

You may have heard of (BCAA) or Branched Chain Amino Acids. The three essential amino acids are (leucine, isoleucine, and valine) grouped together. This group of amino acids increase muscle growth, decrease muscle soreness, and reduce exercise fatigue. But aside from the training aspect, there is new evidence that shows BCAAs help in maintaining the intestinal barrier function (protecting against leaky gut[81]) and promote intestinal regeneration.

L-glutamine is a conditionally essential amino acid. The body does make it, however, during times of crazy physical exercise, levels are depleted and need to be boosted through food or supplements. Glutamine can minimize the breakdown of muscle, improve protein metabolism, and aid in recovery. Not only is it great for physical training but glutamine is also amazing at healing the gut. It improves intestinal barrier function by regulating tight juncture proteins,[82] which is great in treating leaky gut. It also reduces inflammation and rapidly increases enterocytes. Enterocytes are nutrient-absorbing cells located on the surface of the villi.

I take a hydrolyzed collagen peptide protein drink instead of whey or casein. I find it's more nourishing for the gut and I don't have an upset stomach from it. I have a fuller feeling for longer and it boosts my overall health more than the others. It's just like taking extra collagen. I use a specific product from ATP Science called NoWay™.

My 'I've Been Eating Crap Food and Getting Cravings' Regimen

1. Slippery elm bark

2. Chromium

3. Gymnema

Slippery elm bark is just that: a bark. First, it's most commonly used for its anti-inflammatory purposes and gut healing methods of soothing the irritated tissues of the intestines and colon. It's very fibrous and when combined with water it forms a thick slippery gel. I actually chew the pills in between meals so that it expands in my gut to help stop cravings. And aside from healing the gut, it also aids in balancing blood sugar levels.

Chromium is a mineral and is known to enhance the action of insulin. It helps to metabolize carbs, fat, and proteins. I find that if I take chromium in the morning,

[81] Zhou, H., Yu, B., Gao, J., Htoo, J.K., and Chen, D. (2018). "Regulation of intestinal health by branched-chain amino acids". Anim Sci J., 89(1):3-11. doi:10.1111/asj.12937
[82] Rao, R., and Samak, G. (2012). "Role of Glutamine in Protection of Intestinal Epithelial Tight Junctions." *J Epithel Biol Pharmacol, 5(Suppl 1-M7)*:47–54. doi:10.2174/1875044301205010047

it tends to balance out my blood sugar levels and thus I don't feel the need to reach for a snack bar at 3 p.m.

Gymnema is an herb that's been around for centuries and in Hindi means *destroyer of sugar*. This herb contains gymnemic acid which, when eaten, actually fills the sugar receptors of your taste buds. It increases insulin levels and also may reduce the intestine's ability to absorb sugar, reducing blood sugar.

My 'Traveling Soon and Need to Boost Immunity' Regimen

1. Kakadu plum

2. Ki Immune Defence and Energy Formula.

Kakadu plum is only just starting to gain a wider recognition for its health benefits. It's a small deciduous tree found growing extensively throughout the subtropical woodlands of the Northern Territory and Western Australia. It produces crops of small plum-like fruits. The fruit, in fact, holds the world record for the highest content of vitamin C and is full of antioxidants, folic acid, and iron. It has more antioxidants than blueberries and is high in phytonutrients. Not only is it a great supplement to take, I actually have a Kakadu plum body cream that I use on my skin and also have it in jams and spreads.

Ki has Shitake, astragalus, and olive leaf. As listed earlier, Shitake contains essential B vitamins and compounds that have the ability to reduce inflammation, bad bacteria, and viruses. Astragalus has a powerful anti-fungal protein and has been found to have cancer-preventing properties. Olive leaf is a powerful antioxidant.

My 'Had a Bit to Drink Last Night' Regimen

1. Milk thistle

2. White willow bark

3. Chamomile

Milk thistle is my secret special friend. It only takes a couple of glasses of wine for me to feel sick the next day, and if I'm going out to have a big night (again, only ever happens a few times a year) then this is my go-to. Milk thistle detoxifies the liver and kidneys, so before I have a big night, I'll take a couple pills. It really stops the alcohol from getting in my system too much. It also slows down the effect of the drunkenness. I'll also take one before bed, and then when I wake up in the morning. I feel almost normal again.

While my liver and kidneys are getting cleansed from the milk thistle, I want to dull the headache pain a little and this is where white willow bark comes in. Willow bark is just that, a bark off a willow tree. It's been used for centuries as a pain reliever and is not only good for your boozy headache but might also relieve some of the other aches and pains in your body. It's also great for oily skin, acne, and has been known to aid in the treatment of arthritis. What a little gem.

So, my liver is getting cleansed, and I've sorted the headache situation out. Now it's time to rehydrate. Chamomile has been known to help rehydrate and fast.

Overall, this is just *my* supplement regimen. Everyone is different, and as you can see, I don't need a vitamin D supplement, but other people might. I don't need to supplement with B12; again, other people might. So, you will need to customize your own supplement regimen based on your blood work, as one size doesn't fit all.

Am I crazy about taking my vitamins every day? No. Sometimes I forget, or I'm in a rush or I've run out of something. I just try my best when I can. All I want to do is help maintain a healthy system and cover the foundation of probiotics, multi vitamins/minerals, anti-inflammatories, and super antioxidants.

Chapter 21

The Emotional
Rollercoaster

ho would have thought that going gluten-free would bring up a bag of feelings that can make you happy, sad, angry, depressed, and sometimes even make you question yourself?

I wasn't ready for the emotional roller coaster I was about to go on when I cut out gluten. I had no one to tell me what was going to happen emotionally or physically or to give me some reassurance that this emotional rollercoaster was caused by detoxing from the gluten and that I wasn't bat-shit crazy.

Below is a list of emotions I experienced on my journey. Some people might not experience any of this and others might, so I wanted to share my *not so tough* moments in the hope that it helps other people to know they aren't alone.

My emotional roller coaster looked a little something like this.

Shock

When I was first given the news of my diagnosis at the doctor's office, I think I went into shock. You know the kind where it feels like someone hit you in the face with a baseball bat out of nowhere and you literally just sit there like a stunned goat? Yep, that was me.

After my tests and scans concluded, I went back to the hematologist with my husband for the results. I expected and hoped that somewhere I was leaking blood inside my body and that was the cause of the anemia. That would just be a surgical fix. But when the doctor told me I had celiac disease and my intestines had disintegrated, it seemed as though what was left of my life flashed in front of my eyes. I pictured myself trying to travel and not being able to eat what I wanted. No more bread or food festivals. And the list went on.

While I was in shock, my husband was talking to me, but I was completely oblivious to anything he was saying while these scenes played out in my head.

Up for the challenge

By the time I got home, I was feeling *'I can do this.'* It would be ok. My brother was working on some renovations at my house at the time and I told him the news. He was just as shocked as I was, but I proudly held my chin up and said, *"I'm up for the challenge. I can do this."*

Wrong! That feeling lasted a day until I had to clean out my cupboards and started doing some research. It was at this point I thought I wasn't ever going to be able to eat anything I wanted ever again. All hope went out the window and vanished in an instant.

Depression

After my feeling of *up to the challenge* wore off, I found myself becoming increasingly short-tempered and continuously frustrated. At the time, I didn't know that this was, in part, due to the fact I went cold turkey. I was detoxing from the gluten like a drug addict.

I didn't want to eat out anymore and when I did, I was frustrated at not being able to eat what I wanted. I got sick of having very plain food and paying top dollar for it when I could cook something better at home.

Despite my husband being supportive in every way, I was such a bitch to him at times and boy, did I have some tantrums. My body started to go down the shit-chute along with my mind. I was constantly sick. I had clear liquid dripping from my nose like a tap. My skin felt like it was shedding off my body and I constantly wanted to claw at my face.

What probably made it worse was that I didn't just go straight for all the gluten-free alternative food; I knew about the bad additives they contained. So, I simply ate meat, vegetables, salad, and fish. A paleo diet, I guess you could say, not that there's anything wrong with that style of eating. I think it's great. I just wasn't ready for it. I had no energy, no ability to concentrate, and no motivation to try and be creative with meals. At times I think I looked like the crazy old cat lady from *The Simpsons*.

The combination of looking like shit, feeling like shit, and thinking like shit made it so hard to come to grips with it all. I had always been a happy go-lucky person and now every day when I got out of bed, it felt like I was pushing a boulder uphill.

Embarrassment

Around the three- to four-month mark, my body's physical symptoms luckily started to give me a break. But just when I thought things were going to get better, the embarrassment stepped in. I was always an eat-what-I-want-when-I-want person. I was never the *hard work* guest when it came to food. But now I felt like I was one of *those people*; you know, the ones that constantly whine about food.

I didn't want to go out to friends' houses for meals when they invited me as I felt like it put them out trying to think of what to cook for me. It was particularly hard in a group situation because I would have to be the center of focus for the meal. If anyone asked what a particular dish was, the response would be, *"It's gluten-free because Jodie has celiac disease."* Friends also didn't fully understand about cross-contamination or hidden gluten, so scrutinizing their cooking methods was rude, but what do you do? It's hard to have the conversation with your friend who invites you over for dinner and explain to them not only what you can't eat, but also how they have to be careful in preparing it.

I was invited to a dinner with some neighbors who knew I was a celiac. I brought an entrée and they cooked the mains. When we sat down they were so gracious, explaining how they had googled gluten-free. They were so proud of what they made. They really went to a lot of effort and even bought special ingredients. When I saw the tabbouleh on the table I was so excited and said *"Gosh, gluten-free tabbouleh! I love tabbouleh."* They looked at me puzzled and said, *"Is tabbouleh not gluten-free usually?"* I replied that it usually contains cous-cous, and at that point it dawned on them. They were so disappointed and worried because I came so close to being glutened, yet I felt bad for them; they went to so much effort, and now they were worried. It then became a little awkward, disappointing for everyone, and needless to say very embarrassing for me.

Exhaustion

Along with everything else I had to deal with in my life at the time, I was exhausted by constantly having to think of what I was going to eat every day. I was tired of reading labels and I was drained by planning all my meals in advance, thinking of where I was going next and what I had to take just in case I couldn't find something to eat.

Now I had all this extra work. I felt like my happy-go-lucky, spontaneous way of life had literally just gotten up and flown out the damn window.

I was mostly exhausted by people who didn't understand what I was going through. I wasn't after sympathy by any means, but I was tired of telling people I was celiac and having them stand there eating the baguette they randomly picked up for lunch and tell me that this wasn't hard.

Realization

It was at the six-month mark that my husband gave me a kick up the butt hard enough to jolt me right out of my depressed, embarrassed, and exhausted state of mind. At this point there was nothing I could do except come to the realization that this was going to be my life from then on. It felt like a weight lifted off my shoulders once I finally realized I had control issues and was struggling to accept this. I no longer had a choice. I'd had a choice with everything else in life and now with this I didn't. Once this realization set in, I started to feel more open minded about what the future might hold and had to just 'go with it.'

Clarity

I spent my life in the corporate world but always wanted to write a book. From there, the idea to create The GF Hub was born. There was a moment of clarity when I decided that this was what I wanted to do with my life. I wanted to educate people around inflammation and break the norm of just another person advocating gluten-free. I wanted to create a movement, a world, a hub, and a sense of community around this disease. I wanted to create a place filled with all the information that I needed when I was diagnosed. A central meeting point for us.

I started writing this book and developing the GF HUB website. I wanted to shout to the world that simply going gluten-free wasn't going to cut it and I wanted to share what I'd learned. The Hub is in the early stages and still has a long way to go, but it's my passion.

236

Discovery

At this point I'm really learning about all sorts of new foods, ingredients, and styles of cooking. I was always passionate about food, but now I'm embracing the fun, discovery part of living a gluten-free lifestyle. From teff to bone broth to coconut aminos and beyond, there seems to be a never-ending list of new ingredients to work with to create sumptuous food that not only tastes good but is gut-nourishing.

Unity

Once I jumped on Instagram and Facebook and started Googling '*gluten-free groups*,' I discovered the network of amazing people out there. I learned how to bake bread from scratch from a Facebook group called 'Gluten-Free Sourdough Bread' and have made a new network of online friends.

I went to my first gluten-free expo in Brisbane, Australia. It was very small, but I loved speaking to different people and hearing their stories. I stopped by a stand called *Teff Tribe* and a young man and woman were behind a counter filled with all these trendy boxes of teff-related products. I had heard of teff before but had not actually experimented with it yet. I approached the counter, interested in hearing more about their product as I had actually seen it on the shelf of my local store. She told me of their story of how and why they developed this product, and gave me a free box to try.

I had some feel-good vibes going on as I walked away from their stall and on to another where I met Ilona Wilson who runs *Loni's Allergy Free.* We had a great chat about the books she had for sale, and she kindly shared her story.

She is a qualified food scientist, food intolerance sufferer, a lover of food who hates to miss out, and is passionate about home cooking with fresh ingredients. She is a wife who suffers from multiple food intolerances and is mum to three. Her family suffers from lactose intolerance and anaphylactic allergies to nuts, eggs, and seafood. She understands how tricky it can be to navigate meals and cater for multiple allergies and intolerances.

Her range of five cookbooks contain delicious recipes that are free from wheat, gluten, corn, yeast, dairy, egg, peanuts, tree nuts, tomato, sesame seeds, and seafood. You can check out more here.

I told Loni about the book I was writing and the Hub, and she kindly gave me a set of her books to keep for myself along with a special apron. Her intention was not to get free publicity but to share a common value between authors.

I was so stunned at everyone's generosity and community spirit and felt like I might be able to find a place in this new world.

My dear husband had bought me a gluten-free cooking class voucher as a Christmas present. It just so happened to be at the most renown Thai restaurant and cooking school on the Sunshine Coast of Australia called *The Spirit House*. This place is so busy that it actually took me six months to get into an available class. Again, I was surrounded by lots of people who all shared a common value and I met a lovely new friend there who is also a celiac. Wow, my first celiac friend!

After getting myself out there and speaking to people about celiac disease, I found myself meeting the most amazing people and hearing interesting stories just like mine.

I'd found a sense of unity in my new world.

Peace

Now in my fourth year of being diagnosed celiac I have finally found peace with it all. Peace within myself, my family, my friends, and also my new career change in life. I don't worry so much anymore when I can't eat something I want. I have become adept with my new way of eating, and the more time goes on, the easier this all becomes.

Perhaps you might share one or more of these emotional experiences? Perhaps you don't, and you're reading this, laughing at my expense? For many people who have been suffering at the hand of celiac disease complications, achieving a diagnosis may have been the best news they heard. For me, I wanted to share my experience where this caught me by surprise and at first was a curse, not a cure.

New Opportunities

Many of the suppliers of amazing gluten-free food like Monica Topliss have been diagnosed with this condition themselves, and without it, may never have gone on to create amazing products, books, and helpful that can change the world.

Maybe you have a flare for cooking and can write a new gluten-free cookbook, maybe you might develop so much knowledge in the field of health you might become a nutritionist, or maybe you might create the next best food product to curve our insatiable desires?

You never know what amazing new opportunities might arise from this situation, who you might meet, and how your life can change.

Chapter 22

FAQ

(or an interview with myself)

*B*eing celiac does come up in conversation one way or another with new people, and I always get asked the same questions over and over again. I don't mind this at all as I feel explaining it to them is only going to bring about more awareness to celiac disease and gluten intolerance. It seems nowadays nearly anyone I speak to knows of someone in our situation. I never knew anyone with celiac disease before my diagnosis that I could talk to or ask questions after I was diagnosed. I thought it would be fun, and perhaps a little bit interesting, to list the common questions I get asked and answer them in an interview with myself.

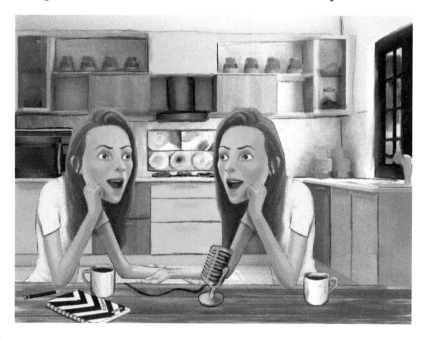

eosFAQ (or an interview with myself)

What do I miss most?

Bread! OMG I miss bread like there is no tomorrow. That crunchy, chewy exterior from an ancient grain sourdough with that soft, cheese-hole interior. There are a few artisan bakers close by where I live and every Friday I call in and grab a fresh traditional sourdough loaf and bring it home to my husband. On occasion I have pulled it out of the bag and had a massive sniff to try and inhale the flavors through my nose but then reality hit me, that's probably not a good idea. Sometimes I've even asked myself, *What would happen if I took a bite, just chewed a little to taste, then spit it out and wash my mouth out?* Short answer: stupid idea!

I just have to sit there and watch my husband slather it with our favorite French d'Affinois double cream brie, then devour it with what looks like orgasmic delight across his face while he groans in satisfaction. Yes, it just sucks not being able to eat bread anymore. I have just experimented with making gluten-free sourdough and although it's nice, I don't think it will ever match up to wheat, but in saying that, I'm sure there are some amazing artisan bakers around the world who could really rival wheat with their creations and I can't wait to try it one day.

What's the hardest part about being celiac?

The hardest part for me is traveling and not being able to live freely anymore. I feel like my spontaneity and the ability to experiment with food is gone. I can't sample food that's held out in front of restaurants anymore. I can't eat everything at a buffet anymore. I can't take the chance and try random foods off the streets in a non-English speaking country. I used to love looking at a menu in Swedish or Arabic, languages I can't speak, and picking something randomly with a point of a finger and getting a surprise when the meal comes out. I used to go to an Italian restaurant so often that my husband and I had eaten pretty much everything off the menu. After a while, when we went in, we weren't presented with menus anymore; the owner would just whip up whatever he felt like for us. So that would be the hardest part now, having to check, double check, and calculate my dining in advance.

Have I ever cheated and eaten gluten knowingly?

Absolutely not. I can say that with such conviction and I'm proud of it! If I was only gluten intolerant, I'd probably be cheating all the time. I'd rather eat something I want to enjoy the moment and put up with not being able to poo for a week. But with celiac, to me it's just non-negotiable. I want to have children and I want to be healthy. I was sick enough with anemia and my fertility problems, and that coupled with the fear of cancer and premature death is enough to ensure I will never ever cheat!

Would I consider taking a pill or vaccine so I can eat what I want?

Short answer: no! Long answer: I don't agree with drugs at the best of times. It doesn't make sense to me to take chemicals to give me the ability to eat something I'm not supposed to eat. You might be thinking, what about taking it when dining out or traveling to mitigate the risk of accidental gluten exposure? To be honest, I think it will take a long time before we will ever get the results of long term studies of these concoctions for me to feel safe taking it. I'd rather rely on my 'E-3 advanced digestive enzymes' that can help with gluten exposure.

How do I deal with the Christmas holidays and similar events?

I do all the cooking! In saying that, though, whenever my family gets together, I've always liked doing the cooking. So, at Christmas time I make everything gluten-free including the gravy. For the appetizers, I have some fresh artisan bread or crackers sitting separately that people can have; otherwise, everything is gluten-free. I'm very lucky to have a family that supports me and they are mostly happy with whatever I make as long as they don't have to cook.

Do I find certain seasons harder than others?

Yes! I struggle in winter. The days are shorter and cold. I don't like shopping at night in the cold much and I'm always craving hearty food like lasagnas, stews, and so on. I tend to crave carbs more in winter. Summer is always the best for me. I bust out the acai bowls for breakfast, salads for lunch, and lean proteins for dinner. I find the range of food I want is more broad and easier to work with in summer than in winter.

Why don't I mention children and celiac disease in my book?

I don't have children so I have no authority on what that might be like and what to do. I must admit it's been quite challenging dealing with myself let alone children who have celiac. So I certainly have much respect and admiration for the people out there who do. I think it would make a good next book so stay tuned in a few years' time.

Do you get sick from accidental gluten exposure now?

Yes, unfortunately. Having completely detoxed from gluten, I do get quite sick at the smallest amount whereas I never used to before. I get a very swollen belly, so much so you would think I was nine months pregnant. Then the narcolepsy sets in. I feel like I'm about to fall asleep immediately no matter where I am. My brain feels like it's shutting down and I yawn every three seconds. I usually want to go and try to sleep it off for a while. For the next few days, I feel just so lousy, tired, and unmotivated. After about three days or so of pushing through, I'll come out good.

What's the most embarrassing moment I've had so far?

Quite a few actually. They usually began with me tip-toeing around a menu to find something to order and then my husband blurting out, *"She has a disease!"* Bloody bastard, I could kill him every time he does that. But it does tend to break the ice and win the waitress or waiter over.

I did get stuck at a Japanese restaurant once. Whatever it was I ate really hit me hard; so hard that I was running around like a chicken without its head to find the bathroom. When I did, and it was occupied, I actually contemplated violating the gardens behind the restaurant! *I was that sick!* The fear of getting caught in the bushes gave me the motivation to beat on the door to the bathroom like a raving lunatic, yelling at the person to get out while holding my bum cheeks closed with one hand and waddling like a duck.

What's my most confusing moment?

Making beef stroganoff for my mother when she was sick. As you are probably aware, when making stroganoff, you flour the beef cubes then fry them off. I knew I wasn't going to be eating this meal and had made it with normal wheat flour, but halfway through cooking it, I got the swollen stomach and narcolepsy feeling. I had to lay down on the couch and sleep it off. I think I was breathing in the flour when I was tossing it around to coat it. You might be laughing at me for this one, but I actually didn't think that was going to be an issue. Turns out it is, so I don't handle flour anymore.

Do I find any major differences now to before I was celiac?

Yes, obviously! I don't have anemia anymore and my fertility is much better. But overall, I think the main difference is that I used to get migraines quite often, weekly actually. I always thought they were because of the car accident I had when I was 16 and the tissue damage I have in my neck. My neck would get tight, in the same place over and over again, and I'd get a migraine. But weirdly enough, I don't suffer from the neck spasms or migraines as much as I used to. So, this could be something that was something attributed to the gluten that I had no idea about.

What's a 'feel good' moment that's come out of being celiac diagnosed?

Not long after I was diagnosed, my brother was visiting. One morning I felt like pancakes. I had never made pancakes before as I'd only ever eaten them at my mother's house and she always made them. Again, not something I ever really craved but did after I was diagnosed. As I was trying to look up recipes, my brother strolled into my kitchen, pulled out my buckwheat flour, baking powder, vanilla extract, eggs, cinnamon, and rice milk and whipped up the most flavorful gluten-free pancakes right there for me. I did enjoy this feel-good brother/sister moment but admit I also felt a little pathetic that my older brother had to teach me how to make pancakes.

Chapter 23

Our Experiences —
Chats with Some Other Celiacs and Gluten-Sensitive People

There is only so much you can learn from books and I read a ton of them. They are mostly written from the perspective of the author with their opinions and experiences (mine included) so I felt like I was only getting one point of view when reading them.

I didn't know anyone with celiac where I could bounce around ideas or ask questions so I had to get out of my comfort zone and hit the forums to find out about how celiac disease affects others. I wanted to know their tips and tricks, what happens to them when they eat gluten, was getting diagnosed a relief, or did they find it hard like myself? I mostly wanted to know how being celiac or NCGS changed their life. It was time for me to connect with others and not feel so alone in this.

After reading their responses, I felt for the first time like I was not being overly-dramatic about my situation. It was nice to know that my frustrations were shared by so many other people. I found their stories to be quite interesting and wanted to share them in this book. I want you to be able to hear not just my own experiences with celiac disease but others too. Our lives are changed forever by this disease and no one person has all the answers.

Hopefully, there are some elements here that you can relate to and, let's face it, we all want to feel connected or understood in some way. It's nice to know you're not alone.

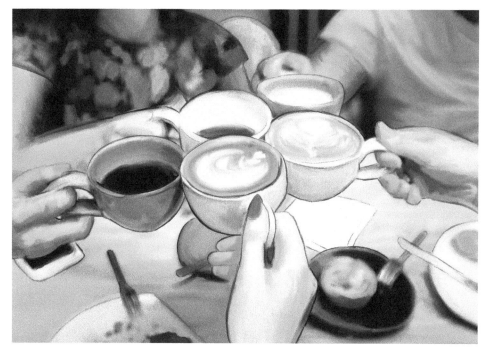

Please note some responses have been edited for clarity.

What do you find is the hardest part of being celiac?

Amy from Adelaide, Australia says:

"The hardest part about being Coeliac is that even though there is much greater awareness now of what it is, there is still a lack of understanding about just how careful we have to be with our food. Cross contamination poses the greatest risk, as despite our own personal efforts to maintain a 100% gluten-free diet, we can be caught out when other people prepare our food or when it is mislabeled. I often have friends offer to cook for me or cater for me at parties and they are shocked when I send them the guidelines for how to safely prepare my food. I find it very difficult to trust other people to get it right."

Sarah from North Carolina, USA says:

"Eating on the go has been challenging. Losing the inability to just eat anything makes it so that there's never the freedom to not worry about having enough or safe food to eat.

The social implications of celiac are also tough. People often like to try and accommodate my gluten-free diet. For example, friends or distant family will go out of their way to make something gluten-free. But it often puts me in a difficult position given my sensitivity. While I don't want to admit I don't trust these people, the reality is, I don't! It's not their fault, but I have a very precise way of ensuring no cross-contamination that somebody who doesn't do it regularly could easily get it wrong. Some of the hardest situations to navigate are when I'm offered food from these people and I need to decide whether to politely decline or just risk eating it."

Anett from Hungary says:

"For me the hardest part always was to eat out and find places to eat during my travels. The hotel industry is getting better at paying attention to guests who have special diets, but cross-contamination is still a huge issue and I find that people don't really get that, or they think you are overreacting. Keeping up with the changes in the food industry (new products, changed ingredients) can be challenging as well."

Chloe from East England, United Kingdom says:

"I don't like being perceived as fussy when I go out to eat and I also find it really difficult when I have to triple check if the food presented to me is indeed gluten-free. It has paid off though as recently I was almost served normal chocolate cake! Additionally it is hard to be spontaneous as I worry about cross contamination in restaurants and when my friends try hard but just forget about using the same spoon etc. then I have to refuse the food. I miss certain foods, but it is the fear of getting accidentally poisoned which is the worst part of the disease."

Judy from Queensland, Australia says:

"Eating with a new acquaintance, relation or workmate. I get edgy at someone's house when they go to use the same chopping board or serving utensils as the non-gluten-free food. It is embarrassing when asking for my food to be separately prepared, plated and/or care taken. I almost feel that people who don't know me will be rolling their eyes as a lot of people eat GF so don't always understand the difference between choice and CD. My close friends and family are understanding."

Erika from Lisbon, Portugal says:

"The hardest part of being Celiac is not having the liberty to eat out in safety. Food has been a part of social life for centuries and with the limitation that I have eating out, it's hard. It's hard because I can no longer eat my favourite foods. Because most of the times I eat in fear, knowing that I might get sick any time afterwards. It's hard explaining myself in a restaurant, both to the staff and also to my family and friends, about the reasons why I cannot eat. It's hard when I travel and I don't have safe options and I live off sandwiches and fruit for a week or two, with no option for a hot meal anywhere. It's hard that I have to plan family vacations based on my restriction and the possibilities for eating.

Sara (Portuguese) living in the United Arab Emirates, Dubai says:

"For me, the hardest part of being Celiac is the social side of it. Coming from a Mediterranean family where everything revolves around food, big family gatherings or having dinner out with friends are events that I usually dread.

Being a flight attendant was not a smart choice of job as well! Having to scavenge my way through the world is not easy mainly when I fly to destinations in Asia or Africa where there is not any awareness about Celiac disease. Also I always need to carry my own food everywhere. I can never rely on finding food if I am flying to an unknown place."

What are your tips and tricks for eating out?

Sarah from New South Wales, Australia says:

"My tips and tricks for eating out include research! You can never do enough research before eating out. I will first look for other coeliac's recommendations (Facebook groups for coeliacs or on forums). I will then call the restaurant or send them a Facebook message to identify if they cater for 'gluten-free' or for 'coeliacs with no cross contamination' as there is a difference. When I am travelling I do all this research and 'star' the safe places on Google Maps which I can access on the road to see which places are close to me."

Kellie from Queensland, Australia says:

"Research, research, research! I spend a lot of time online, particularly if we are going away on holidays. I start with TripAdvisor and their top 20 recommended places to eat. I then Google the actual restaurant/food place to look

at their menu. I also rely on the Facebook page *Coeliac Disease Support Group Australia*. I read reviews left by other people and I also add a lot of reviews myself. I have some very extensive spreadsheets now on various destinations. For my local favourites, once we have found a place that is suitable, reliable and knowledgeable, we tend to stick with it."

Jasmine from Minnesota, USA says:

"Before I eat anywhere, I look it up on the app *Find Me Gluten-free* and check its ratings and reviews. I will also google them for more information or call if needed. Once at the restaurant, I will ask for a gluten-free menu and question the waitress / waiter about the precautions taken. If I feel safe ordering, I will make sure they note my order as a gluten allergy (even though it isn't an allergy). I have found that is a good way to get people to understand it."

Bianca from New South Wales, Australia says:

"Reach out on social media to see where other Celiacs in your area like to eat. I am a part of multiple Facebook groups, and have an active Instagram account dedicated to following Celiac hashtags and other Celiacs in my area. I have found that this has shown me many places I wouldn't have guessed would have safe options, including my local Japanese place that makes their own GF teriyaki!"

Amy from Adelaide, Australia says:

"I carry business sized cards with me that explain my condition and some guidelines for preparing food safely without cross contamination. This helps the servers communicate to the kitchen what my needs are. But my best tip is to ask the server to show the card to chef and then get the chef's recommendation on what they can prepare for me, versus trying to choose something off the menu that I think will be safe. The chef knows best what their preparation environment is like, and I've learned not to be fussy. Whatever the chef thinks is the safest is what I order."

Chloe from East England, United Kingdom says:

"I always try to find restaurants which have naturally gluten-free food. Usually I chose Vietnamese places as I know most of the menu will be naturally gluten-free plus I like the taste! When I lived in the US there were plenty of fabulous Mexican restaurants too.

Otherwise, I would try to plan where to go in advance or have a look at the menu if I'm not able to choose (a friend's birthday or something) at least before getting there so that I know what I might like or what I could easily ask to be adapted for me. I have learnt not to be fussy and just accept anything which is safe, however this does make eating out less pleasurable than it used to be."

Avah (13 years old) from Illinois, USA says:

"Look online before going to the restaurant. Reading through the menu so you have an idea of what gluten-free options you will have. This helps me have an idea of what I can eat and what I won't be able to get. I feel less upset if I know before I get to the restaurant."

Sara (Portuguese) living in the United Arab Emirates, Dubai says:

"I think I will never lose that fear of eating out... It's always a Russian roulette, especially when you visit new places.

*However and because I do it on a weekly basis here are my tips & tricks: **try to go for celiac friendly certified places.***

In Europe, most Celiac Associations have certified restaurants where the menu and the staff is celiac aware and oriented. For example, in Portugal, the Portuguese Celiac Organization has a page dedicated to eating out with a list of bakeries, hotels, restaurants that make our lives much, much easier.

*If you cannot find certified places, go to places that have gluten-free items on the menu and explain them your disease. Explaining celiac disease is not easy at all. People just want to know if you are going to have an **anaphylactic shock** which doesn't happen in my case. So try to explain them how important it is for your food to be prepared gluten-free in a contamination free environment even if you are not going to have a shock.*

Try to look up places online or follow a few celiac blogs. If you're invited to a party or a dinner out check out the menu of the place online and don't be afraid to call them just to double check if they can accommodate you.

If you are going abroad and especially if you don't speak the language, check a few celiac travel blogs beforehand (I love the Legal Nomads) and don't forget to take some gluten-free restaurant cards with you. Also try to do a little research on local food in order to understand what might be the threat for you as a celiac.

Write down the names in the local language and take pictures with you in case you need to point! Also, if you can stay somewhere with a kitchen (apartment hotel, for example) that will make your life much easier. Don't expect people to fully understand your disease, but never be afraid to ask questions and when in doubt, don't eat. You can always rely on fruits and water, at least for a day!"

How do you cope with being celiac in your family?

Kellie from Queensland, Australia says:

"I am also a vegetarian and have been for many years (30), whereas the Coeliac diagnosis is only about 2 years old. I am used to cooking two meals for our family. Gradually though I have incorporated more gluten-free meals into their lives too, without taking over completely. I will often make my meal as a main meal for myself but as a side dish for the rest of my family, which I will serve with meat for them. Apart from tofu they are happy with that."

Sarah from New South Wales, Australia says:

"When I'm cooking, I cook 100% gluten-free for the family to reduce the risk of any cross-contamination. If we are having bread I make sure this is completely separate to the preparation area. When we eat out, the family can each order what they want but in this case I have to make sure no little gluten hands or gluten kisses go anywhere near me! It can be a challenge teaching kids to not share their food with me or put their fork or hands on my plate."

Heather from Texas, USA says:

"Myself and two of my children are celiac. My husband and other child are intolerant. Over the years I have subbed our regular meals with a gluten-free option. I cook 6-7 days a week and we rarely eat out. Pinterest is a huge help with recipes and reviews. We do a lot of meat, rice, vegetables and fruit. I have mastered some old family recipes that I craved and they turned out great. It takes time and patience, but you can become confident cooking and baking gluten-free."

Jasmine from Minnesota, USA says:

"Since being diagnosed, I have been the only one in my household to be gluten-free. I have my own cupboard of food, cutting boards, toaster, etc. and everybody knows not to contaminate my things or shared food items. Gluten-free food has

come a long way and can taste very good, so if I do make gluten-free meals for my family they eat whatever it is that I made."

Erika from Lisbon, Portugal says:

"I am lucky to have a very understanding husband who eats what I cook at home. Outside our home he can eat whatever he wants, but our home keeps gluten-free. Our family members know of my situation and accept it that when they come to our house, all the food will be gluten-free. We don't risk contamination in the house."

Amy from Adelaide, Australia says:

"I am the only Coeliac in my household. Both my husband and my daughter eat gluten containing foods regularly. If I'm preparing food for myself and my family, it's always 100% gluten-free and they eat what I eat. But I also prepare food that contains gluten for them (that I don't eat) and we are just very careful about cleanliness in the kitchen, separate sections of the fridge/cupboards for gluten-free foods and separate pots/pans for my food. It took some getting used to, but now that we are in the habit of being careful it just comes naturally."

Sara (Portuguese) living in the United Arab Emirates, Dubai, says:

"The first months were quite challenging but eventually everything just fell into place. I still lived with my family when I was diagnosed so the whole family mindset had to change. My sister was also diagnosed so immediately my parents understood the importance of changing our kitchen habits.

Gluten-free and non gluten-free food was separated, new tools were bought, we bought a new toaster and new containers for the food. It was hard for them to understand a few concepts about cross contamination but the hardest was the explain to my grandmothers that we could not eat some of our favorite dishes anymore ☹ up until today (and almost 5 years have passed) they still call us in advance every time we go there for dinner just to make sure that what they prepared is suitable for us. Bless them.

At the moment I live with my husband in Dubai and he's the absolute best. He is a great cook so he tries to adapt everything to my diet. KFC style chicken, Arabic dishes, classical Portuguese comfort food, you name it, he finds a way to cook it for me."

What happens when you are accidentally glutened?

Alesha from Queensland, Australia says:

"If I am accidentally glutened, I will be home sick within 4 hours with stomach pains and an upset stomach. Generally for a week following, I will have a foggy brain, easily lose my train of thought, breakouts and headaches. If it is a large dose of gluten, I will have migraines. My training and work are affected for up to two weeks."

Heather from Texas, USA says:

"My stomach starts burning almost instantly. Within about 30-60 minutes I feel like I am being cut open with [a] razor blade from the inside out. This will last for days. I become incredibly bloated, and will violently throw up along with diarrhea. The next three days my lower back is so sore along with joint pain, brain fog, and a migraine like headache."

Bianca from New South Wales, Australia says:

"If I am accidentally glutened, I don't seem to get the major gastrointestinal effects that others have. Instead, I have intense joint pain. I feel as though I am constantly walking through mud, and all movements are a struggle. With this comes fatigue and the dreaded brain fog."

Chloe from East England, United Kingdom says:

"First off, I get very sharp shooting pain in my stomach and an irresistible urge to eat as many gluten-containing foods as possible within reach. Obviously my rational mind wins and doesn't allow me to gluttonously devour anything which would do me more harm, but the fight is real at that point!

I then become incredibly sleepy to the point where I once fell asleep on an Italian family's dining table after having been assured the crustless quiche was safe!

When I awake which is usually after a considerable time, I feel as though I've been drugged. I'm disorientated, dizzy with a fuzzy head reminiscent of a bad hangover. Processing information becomes next to impossible and I get snappy and sluggish. I will often vomit at this stage as well.

Following on from the initial 48 hour period, I will have a little brain fog leftover but mainly I will experience a constant ache in my joints, especially my wrists and fingers when I type, write or chop. This usually lasts a month or so."

Sarah from New South Wales, Australia says:

"I get really terrible migraines, diarrhea, vomiting and stomach pains for close to a week depending on the severity of how much I've ingested. This sets me back physically up to a few months. As soon as you damage your villi it can take months for them to heal! Mentally this also sets me back a long way - it's so disheartening to find out someone else has made a choice about your health and decided to either not disclose some sort of cross-contamination that is taking place in the kitchen of their restaurant, or not take your coeliac questions seriously and lied about a source of cross-contamination or certain ingredients being included in the dish."

Avah (13 years old) from Illinois, USA says:

"If I accidentally get gluten I feel sad. I usually get a stomach ache and a headache. I then reflect on what I ate to figure out where the gluten came from. Usually it's from cross contamination."

Amy from Adelaide, Australia says:

"I am a very lucky Coeliac in that I am asymptomatic when it comes to short term exposure to gluten. I only experience symptoms when exposed longer term to gluten (depression, hair loss, malnourishment). If I am accidentally glutened I am sometimes unaware of it. If I am aware of it, I make absolutely certain that I remain 100% gluten-free and take extra caution in the following weeks as I know the damage has been done, despite not necessarily feeling it."

Do you have any significant positive differences in your life now, compared to pre-diagnosis?

Bianca from New South Wales, Australia says:

"I have so much more energy! Right before I was diagnosed, I would spend all weekend napping. I would wake up to eat breakfast, and then fall asleep again. At work, I would need to head home at 3pm each day because I couldn't stay awake. Waking up before 8.30 was a struggle. Now, I am up at 7am and spend my

weekends walking and hiking. The other impact is that I am now so much more conscious of what I eat. I don't find myself craving processed foods as much, and vegetables are a huge part of my diet now. That definitely helps with my energy levels too!"

Kellie from Queensland, Australia says:

"I am definitely a much better cook! Having to read labels and find recipes was daunting to start with but now I love it. My spice rack has gone from basil and pepper to an amazing assortment of spices. In fact, I need another spice rack to cope! I am cooking with ingredients I had never heard of before and experimenting more. I am lucky that my family is understanding and happy to eat most things. If I make a recipe now and it's not great I can usually think of ways to improve it. That would never have happened in the past! I find I am much more creative."

Sarah from New South Wales, Australia says:

"There are many significant positives in my life now. My health has never been better, I'm happier and no longer get migraines weekly. My fitness has improved by a long way - before I was diagnosed I was quite malnourished and fatigued, and now I'm able to participate at work, in a fitness class or conversation without being exhausted feeling like I'm going to fall asleep mid-conversation."

Sarah from North Carolina, USA says:

"I was diagnosed with an unknown form of juvenile arthritis at the age of 8. It progressed pretty significantly over time and I ended up on injectable biologics/low-dose chemo at 11 years old. This rotation of various drugs continued throughout my teens as my symptoms increased. I had inflammation in almost every joint in my body. Freshman year at college, I started having stomach issues and lost most of my hair in about 4 months' time. I had never had these symptoms... at least not until I started drinking beer :) It only took a few months of symptoms to get me to see a pediatric GI, who immediately tested for celiac (it was positive). I went gluten-free and my arthritis has been in "remission" ever since. I am drug free for almost 5 years! My doctors are pretty confident that my arthritis was a primary symptom of undiagnosed celiac for all those years. So... I DEFINITELY have MAJOR positive differences now compared to pre diagnosis :) And - all my hair grew back!"

Heather from Texas, USA says:

"I wanted to die! I was sick for 6 months and the Dr. I had been seeing told me I was crazy and making up my symptoms for attention. I would be in so much pain at night I would be sobbing. My husband felt helpless. With the help of a new Dr. I was diagnosed relatively quickly and was feeling better within a few weeks. Healing kept coming. At the one year mark of being gluten-free, dairy started to bother me. We are now a gluten-free, dairy free family. Going on 4 years. It's not always easy. I try to make life for my kids as normal as possible for them. This can easily cripple you and socially isolate you. So hang in, keep pushing on. You can do it too and never let this hold you back in life."

Tayler from Ohio, USA says:

"Heck yes! I am less anxious, happier, and overall more comfortable physically and mentally. I spend significantly less time in the bathroom or curled up in my bed in pain and more time enjoying my life. I welcomed my diagnosis because for years I had no answers to my digestive issues. Finally getting a concrete answer on how I can stop what felt like my body failing me was a blessing."

Danielle (8 years old) from Missouri, USA says:

"I have gained weight and height and my family says color too!"

"I do not look like a "typical" Coeliac, in that I am overweight, so it took a long time for me to get a diagnosis. I went to my doctor in 2016 complaining of depression, hair loss, fatigue, low iron and low vitamin D and after numerous tests a different doctor (who is Coeliac herself) suggested we test for it just in case. Sure enough, the antibodies showed up in my blood test and an endoscopy confirmed it and I got my diagnosis. Since then, my depression lifted within a month of eating 100% gluten-free and my iron levels have slowly improved over the last two years. The diagnosis felt like a life sentence at the beginning, but I quickly adapted to the new way of life and now it doesn't bother me at all!"

Avah (13 years old) from Illinois, USA says:

"I feel happier than I did when I ate gluten. I have grown in height and weight. I used to be the shortest in my school and in the negative for my percentage in

height and weight. Now I'm still short but the positive percentage wise for height and weight."

Anett from Hungary says:

"Yes, many positive differences. All my symptoms went away that were causing me daily struggle. I also learnt a lot about other allergies/ intolerances and I try to help other people with my experiences and knowledge."

Chloe from East England, United Kingdom says:

"I have a much greater empathy for anyone with a particular illness, especially those which are not well understood by the public as it isn't a case of being fussy, it's a case of a month of pain in my case, with some people having even more severe reactions.

Personally, I do quite like being able to refuse foods on a medical basis rather than just appearing fussy. For example when people bring cake into work. I only like chocolate cake, but I know it would look rude to refuse to join in so I'm grateful that my disease can act as my legitimate excuse!"

Sara (Portuguese) living in the United Arab Emirates, Dubai, says:

"Before being diagnosed I was pretty much a silent celiac. I was only tested because my sister was diagnosed. The only symptoms I had from my teenager years onwards were eczema, cold sores and a persistent iron deficiency. Until I started the diet I never understood that they were related to gluten. Being able to have more energy and a better looking skin gave me a confidence boost and I am really grateful to have found the cause."

Chapter 24

Final Notes
and Takeaways

Thank you for reading my book. I hope you have enjoyed it and my babbling makes some sense to you. A few final takeaway points to remember for your journey.

1. Always keep a healthy snack alternative close by at work, in your handbag, in your car, etc.

2. Avoid anything that has modified starch and be wary of additives.

3. Keep your cheat sheets on your phone or printed out in your wallet/purse.

4. Be kind to people when they offer you food that has gluten in it; they've either forgotten or just really don't know. Don't get angry at your families' ignorance when they say, *"Surely just a little bit won't hurt."* You're going to have that happen more than once.

5. Get your emergency kit in place. You will be exposed to gluten more than once moving forward in your life so you might want to think about your plan to deal with it.

   - What supplements do you need?

   - What is going to be your action plan?

6. Continue to do your research (like reading this book) and connect with others. The more you know, the easier life will be.

7. Spread the word about celiac disease. If we make enough noise together, we may be able to help others achieve an earlier diagnosis, and they won't suffer as long as we have.

Overall, nobody should know your body better than you. You're the one who has to live with it for the rest of your life, not some doctor and not some internet forum. Your body is your temple, your home, you are responsible for it and when it expires or fails you are not getting a new one.

Be kind to your body but also know that life is short. Too short. If you want to eat corn, go eat corn. If you want to drink booze, go drink booze. Just do the best you can and find *your* balance

If you can adopt a healthy lifestyle 90% of the time, then you're already doing better than most. Enjoy that other 10%; splurge and have fun. Don't count your calories or your crumbs. If you want a cheat meal, make it a good one. You have to live life and stressing over every little crumb can do your body more harm. This was one of the hardest lessons I had to learn.

Remember to reflect on the positives that can come; maybe there might be a new direction or path your life might take?

Please feel free to reach out to me directly with any questions you may have and if possible, I would greatly appreciate it if you could write a review for me.

But my most honest request to you and the whole purpose of this book is:

> "Remember, a simple diet switch, is not what it seems, please be mindful of gluten-free products and make better choices. You deserve to be happy and healthy."

Thank you for joining me on my gluten-free journey, all the very best with yours. Let's stay in touch.

xx,

Jodes

Chapter 25

Resources:
Facebook Groups, Websites, Books and More

Who doesn't love resources? You're armed with all my jargon, thoughts, and experiences but let's direct you to some further stuff that can help you on your journey.

The next few pages will outline:

✓ Facebook groups. *These are groups I'm personally involved in.*

✓ Celiac disease organizations / foundations / centers / programs

✓ Recommended websites. *Blogs and companies I love.*

✓ Apps for mobile phones

✓ Recommended books. *My personal library of reads.*

✓ YouTube videos. *Awesome must-watch educational videos.*

✓ Magazines

✓ Global events

✓ E-number Nasties Cheat Sheets

✓ Comprehensive List of Food Additives to Avoid

Recommended Facebook Groups

Facebook groups are a great resource. I've learned a lot from some groups and they have connected me to such a large network of people. This was super handy considering I knew only one person with celiac disease and I only met her months after I was diagnosed, so initially I felt like I was on my own. I've joined groups in areas that I live in, and also areas that I travel to, like Las Vegas. I've also found out about upcoming events through groups so they have been very handy.

However, like with everything, you need to exercise caution when asking and giving advice on Facebook groups. People can be very opinionated, and I've seen people leave groups because of bullying. It's an unfortunate truth. A lot of people also think they are experts on Facebook and many people use it as a way to exercise some authority, so just be mindful when participating.

Here are my top groups that I'm part of; there are, however, many, many more you can join:

General Global Groups

- The Gluten-Free Hub - Our very own GF Hub group where all are welcome. It's designed as a global group for news, events, research, recipes, and general chit chat.

- Gluten-free Sourdough Baking (This is one of my favorites)

- Celiac Disease

- Gluten-free

- The Gluten-free Blogger Group

- Gluten-free Families

- Dairy, Gluten, Soy Free, Paleo, Organic Allergy Friendly and More

- Celiac Disease and NCGS Support Group

- Gluten-free Travel

- Celiac Travel

- Easy Gluten-Free Recipes

- Gluten-free Living and Recipe Share

- Grub Without Gluten

- Gluten-free and Me

- Life with Celiac Disease

- Women with Celiac - Living Realistically with Celiac Disease

Australia / New Zealand Groups

- Coeliac Disease Support Group Vic, Australia

- Gluten-free New Zealand

- Gluten-free Melbourne

- The Yum Gluten-free Village

- Australia's Gluten and Celiac Support Group
- Gluten-free AU - For Australians Who Can't Eat Gluten
- Gluten-free Vegans Australia
- Gluten-Free & Dairy Free Lifestyle (Australia)

USA Groups

- Gluten-free Las Vegas

Europe Groups

- Gluten-free Italy

UK Groups

- Gluten-free and from the UK

Asia Groups

- Gluten-Free Expats Japan

Celiac Disease Organizations, Foundations, Centers, and Programs

United States

- Boston Children's Hospital Celiac Disease Program childrenshospital.org/centers-and-services/celiac-disease-program

- Center for Celiac Research, Massachusetts General Hospital celiaccenter.org

- The Celiac Disease Center at Columbia University celiacdiseasecenter.columbia.edu

- The Celiac Center at the University of Tennessee utmedicalcenter.org

- Center for Digestive Disease at the University of Iowa uihealthcare.org/celiacdisease

- Mayo Clinic in Minnesota mayoclinic.org/celiac-disease

- The University of Chicago Celiac Disease Center cureceliacdisease.org

- Celiac Disease Foundation celiac.org

- American Celiac Disease Alliance americanceliac.org

- Children's Digestive Health and Nutrition Foundation cdhnf.org

Canada

- Canadian Celiac Association Celiac.ca

Australia

- Coeliac Australia coeliac.org.au

- Gastroenterological Society of Australia gesa.org.au

UK

- Coeliac UK coeliac.org.uk

Recommended Websites

This is a list of my top favorite websites.

- **The Gluten-Free Hub** thegfhub.com

  The Hub will be a place for us to connect, learn, and thrive in the GF world.

- **Dr. Tom O'Bryan** thedr.com/clinical-services

  Dr. Tom O'Bryan is a world leader at the forefront of celiac disease. He has written books, hosts online discussions, provides clinical services for patients, and runs an informative blog.

- **iHerb** iHerb.com

  I love this website for buying not only food but also bath and body products. They have a sorting function that makes it easy to find great gluten-free products. I shop with them regularly and they have given me a code to share with others, which means you will get 5% of your total cart. You can use it as many times as you like for a discount. Here is the code: **AOS6454**. Just simply paste it in the coupon section when you check out.

- **Gluten-free Society** glutenfreesociety.org

  An informative website for doctors and patients about gluten sensitivity.

- **National Foundation for Celiac Awareness** beyondceliac.org

  Beyond Celiac is a website that publishes helpful resources and the latest updates on celiac disease research.

- **Gluten-free Passport** glutenfreepassport.com

  This is a helpful website for international travel resources. It contains guides, dining cards, and a helpful forum.

- **Gluten-free Watchdog** glutenfreewatchdog.org

  This is a great company who tests products labeled gluten-free and blows the whistle on misleading products and companies.

- **Clean Gut Program** cleanprogram.com

  One of my favorite physicians, Dr. Alejandro Junger, has founded the clean gut program, a nutritional cleanse detox and healthy diet program.

- **The Paleo Mom** thepaleomom.com
  Dr. Sarah Ballantyne is a medical biophysicist and has founded this website that centers around nutrition and advice for auto-immune conditions.

Recommended Apps for Cell Phones

Where would we be these days without our trusty little phone? That itty bitty piece of machinery we hold in the palm of our hand holds more technology than a rocket ship sent to the moon! Having some handy apps for on the go makes life just a bit easier. Below are my top rated apps I use regularly.

Find Me Gluten-free findmeglutenfree.com

A global directory for finding gluten-free restaurants.

Gluten-free Restaurant Cards celiactravel.com

An app that has multiple language restaurant cards.

Allergy Eats allergyeats.com

An app to find allergy-centered restaurants throughout the United States.

Fooducate Product Scanner fooducate.com

Dietary tracking app for products within the United States.

The Gluten-free Scanner scanglutenfree.com

USA food product label scanner.

Sift Food Labels siftfoodlabels.com

Another great label scanner. Sift will translate the real ingredients so you know what's in your food and flag any risky ingredients.

Green Kitchen Stories greenkitchenstories.com

These guys have two apps that I love. Green food and deserts. You can set the parameters to remove the recipes with gluten and you're left with a ton of healthy delicious meals.

Recommended Books

Who doesn't love a good book? If only I was going to promote something like *Fifty Shades of Grey* it would make it so much more interesting! But I'm not.

When I was diagnosed, I was finishing a book a week on celiac disease for months and my collection outgrew the bookcase. Not everyone has time to read a million books like I did, so I hope I've done a good job at summarizing a lot of the information into this one. Below are my top picks for recommended books on celiac disease, gluten intolerance, recipes, allergies, and general health from my library.

A little disclaimer here...*some of the links below are affiliate links, meaning— at no additional cost to you—I will earn a commission if you click through and make a purchase.* Please know that I personally own a copy of everything I am recommending and wouldn't recommend it if I didn't believe it be of value to you. The tiny bit of commission helps to pay for the production of this book and also goes to the GF Hub website. I hope you don't mind, and your support is greatly appreciated.

The Autoimmune Fix by Tom O'Bryan

"How to Stop the Hidden Autoimmune Damage That Keeps You Sick, Tired, and Fat Before it Turns Into Disease".

You Can Fix Your Brain by Tom O'Bryan

Just 1 Hour a Week to the Best Memory, Productivity, and Sleep You've Ever Had.

Wheat Belly by William Davis.

Lose the Wheat, Lose the Weight, and Find Your Path Back to Health.

Wheat Belly Cook Book by William Davis.

150 Recipes to Help You Lose the Wheat, Lose the Weight, and Find Your Path Back to Health.

No Grain No Pain by Dr Peter Osborne.

A 30 day diet for eliminating the root cause of Chronic Pain.

Coconut Cures by Bruce Fife.

Preventing & Treating Common Health Problems with Coconut.

Celiac Disease by Peter Green.

Celiac disease is an auto-immune disorder that affects nearly one in every hundred people. Unfortunately, 97 percent remain undiagnosed and untreated.

Health Wars by Phillip Day.

A comprehensive collection of information covering Fluoride to the Sun.

Gluten-freedom by Alessio Fasano.

The Nation's Leading Expert Offers the Essential Guide to a Healthy, Gluten-Free Lifestyle.

Grain Brain by Dr. Perlmutter.

The Surprising Truth about Wheat, Carbs, and Sugar - Your Brain's Silent Killers.

Dissolving Illusions by Roman Bystrianyk and Suzanne Humphries MD.

Disease, Vaccines, and the Forgotten History.

Gluten Is My Bitch by April Peveteaux.

Rants, Recipes, and Ridiculousness for the Gluten-Free.

Jennifer's Way by Jennifer L. Esposito.

My Journey with Celiac Disease—What Doctors Don't Tell You and How You Can Learn to Live Again.

The Gluten-free Revolution by Jax Peters Lowell

Absolutely Everything You Need to Know about Losing the Wheat, Reclaiming Your Health, and Eating Happily Ever After.

The First Year, Celiac Disease by Jules E. Dowler Shepard

Celiac Disease and Living Gluten-Free: An Essential Guide for the Newly Diagnosed.

Celiac Disease for Dummies by Ian Blumer & Sheila Crowe.

Celiac Disease for Dummies is the ultimate reference for people with the disease and their family members

Celiac Disease by Sylvia Llewelyn Bower & Steve Plogsted & Mary Kay Sharrett. *A Guide to Living with Gluten Intolerance.*

Understanding Celiac Disease by Naheed S Ali.

An Introduction for Patients and Caregivers.

The Gluten Connection by Shari Lieberman

How Gluten Sensitivity May Be Sabotaging Your Health - And What You Can Do to Take Control Now.

The G Free Diet by Elisabeth Hasselbeck.

A Gluten-Free Survival Guide.

Gut by Giulia Enders.

The inside story of our body's most under-rated organ.

Promise and Fulfilment by Chris Graeme John Stafferton

Formulas for real bread without gluten.

Minimalist Baker Every Day Cooking by Dana Shultz.

101 Entirely Plant-Based, Mostly Gluten-Free, Easy and Delicious Recipes.

Gluten-Free Artisan Bread in Five Minutes a Day by Jeff Hertzberg & Zoe Francois.

The Baking Revolution Continues with 90 New, Delicious and Easy Recipes Made with Gluten-Free Flours.

Against all Grain by Danielle Walker

Meals Made Simple: Gluten-Free, Dairy-Free, and Paleo Recipes to Make Anytime.

Gluten-Free On A Shoestring by Nicole Hunn

125 Easy Recipes for Eating Well on the Cheap.

201 Gluten-Free Recipe For Kids by Carrie S Forbes.

Chicken Nuggets! Pizza! Birthday Cake! All Your Kids' Favorites - All Gluten-Free!

The Gluten-Free Asian Kitchen by Laura Byrne Russell

In The Gluten-Free Asian Kitchen, food writer Laura B. Russell shows home cooks how to convert the vibrant cuisines of China, Japan, Korea, Thailand, and Vietnam into gluten-free favorites.

The Gloriously Gluten-Free Cookbook by Vanessa Maltin

Spicing Up Life with Italian, Asian, and Mexican Recipes.

Gluten-Free Girl by Shauna James Ahern

How I Found the Food That Loves Me Back... and How You Can Too

The Road to Perfect Health by Brenda Watson

Balance your gut, Heal your body: A modern guide to curing chronic disease.

Gut Solutions by Brenda watson

Natural solutions to your digestive problems.

Recommended YouTube Videos

Aside from books, magazines, and podcasts, sometimes It's just more fun to watch something. Here are a few great videos to get you going, so pour a cup of your favorite drink, sit back, and enjoy. There are many more on the Hub's site – head to **www.thegfhub.com/videos**

Individual Unique Clips:

- **Daily Bread - Can any human body handle gluten?**
  https://www.youtube.com/watch?v=J6JrHteOsll&vl=en

- **Gluten and GMOs, Jeffrey Smith interviews Dr. Stephanie Seneff**
  https://www.youtube.com/watch?v=KVo51yLnohY&feature=emb_logo

- **The McGovern Report**
  https://www.youtube.com/watch?v=xbFQc2kxm9c&list=PLGuUGzhGRw6VuSvXzR9HgDpx9X5rEMH3i&index=2&t=1s

- **Uprooting the leading cause of death:**
  https://www.youtube.com/watch?time_continue=2&v=30gEiweaAVQ&feature=emb_logo

- **Diagnosing Celiac Disease**
  https://vimeo.com/273835130

- **Food for thought:**
  https://www.youtube.com/watch?v=awtmTJW9ic8&t=118s

- **Gluten Explain: What it is and how it affects your heath:**

https://www.youtube.com/watch?v=SMKweZ4tvLo&feature=emb_logo

- **What's with wheat:**

  https://www.youtube.com/watch?v=5wWR4SljdY4&feature=emb_logo

- **Re-structured Meat (This will change the way you look and buy meat forever):**

  https://www.youtube.com/watch?v=kLYnY_BW3Os&list=PLGuUGzhGRw6UHlTenbnJRfZ7UoSuoq-Oi

- **Gut Brain:**

  https://www.youtube.com/watch?v=mioR_WrkRaU&list=PLGuUGzhGRw6WnE4Kb8uUzAEFPgNu1ss-z

- **Should wheat be reclassified as a narcotic:**

  https://www.youtube.com/watch?v=pK09PCAR4Ys&feature=emb_logo

Channels I subscribe to:

- **Dr. Tom O'Bryan:**

  https://www.youtube.com/channel/UCzlefeGh3JA-Nm0jtf9iYoQ

- **Dr. Osborne:**

  https://www.youtube.com/channel/UCoiSo5WDJmRxOf2cqgC7DSg

- **Dr. David Permutter:**

  https://www.youtube.com/channel/UCDRI_UAXxbHyOOjklnA0dxQ

- **The Gerson Institute:**

  https://www.youtube.com/user/gersoninstitute

- **The Institute for Functional Medicine:**

  https://www.youtube.com/user/I4FunctionalMedicine

- **Alejandro Junger:**

  https://www.youtube.com/user/alejandrojunger

- **William Davis:**

https://www.youtube.com/user/wheatbelly

A Must Watch Video

- https://whatswithwheat.com

Recommended Magazines

These are my top favorite magazines to check out. They are always full of tasty recipes, insightful information, and lots of product advertising so you can see what's out in the marketplace.

I often come across the 'aha' moment in magazines when trying to figure out how to make a certain dish. I've even found the best dumpling recipe in a magazine, so to me they are just as valuable as Pinterest. These magazines are from Australia, the United States, and the UK. Most offer a digital subscription thus removing the oceans between countries.

- *Gluten-free & More* glutenfreeandmore.com
- *Gluten-Free Living* glutenfreeliving.com
- *Simply Gluten-Free* simplygluten-free.com
- *Gluten-Free Heaven* freefromheaven.com
- *GFF Magazine* gffmag.com
- *Australian Gluten-Free Life* agfl.com.au
- *Yum Gluten-Free* yumglutenfree.com.au
- *Delight Gluten-Free* delightglutenfree.com
- *Allergic Living* allergicliving.com
- *Paleo Magazine* paleomagazine.com

Global Events

Why not get among others at some events specially designed for celiac disease, gluten intolerance, and the health conscious?

Australia

- *The Gluten-Free Expo* hosted by Coeliac Australia.
  glutenfreeexpo.com.au
- *Free From Show and Allergy Show*
  freefromshow.com.au/about

United Kingdom

- *Coeliac UK - Gluten-Free Food Festival*
  coeliac.org.uk/get-involved/events
- *Glasgow Gluten-Free Food Fair*
  coeliac.org.uk/get-involved/events
- *Coeliac UK - Whales Gluten-Free Show*
  coeliac.org.uk/get-involved/events
- *Wessex Gluten-Free Food Fair*
  coeliac.org.uk/get-involved/events
- *Gluten-Free Industry Day*
  coeliac.org.uk/get-involved/events
- *The Allergy & Free From Show*
  allergyshow.co.uk/london
- *Free From Festival*
  freefromfestival.co.uk

United States

- *Nourished Festival* nourishedfestival.com
- *Living Free Expo* livingfreeexpo.com
- *DC Gluten-free Expo* dcglutenfreeexpo.com
- *International Celiac Disease Symposium* icds2019-paris.com
- *Central PA Gluten-Free Expo* glutenfreeexpopa.com/central-pa/

E-Number Nasties Cheat Sheets

Please visit thegfhub.com/free-stuff to download the available cheat sheets. We've talked about various E-Numbers already in this book and the cheat sheets for these are available on the website there is available:

The Top 12 Food Additives to Avoid:

These are what I consider to be the nastiest of the nasty additives that I try to avoid at all costs.

Food additives, unfortunately, have managed to make their way into so many of our processed foods. They are also labeled differently depending on which country you're living in, so keeping track of what's-what can be quite tricky. In Australia and Europe, additives are labeled with their E-Number classification, whereas in the USA additives are labeled with their technical name.

Additives certainly do not 'add' anything beneficial to your food! Food is supposed to be as nature intended. Additives make the product more shelf stable, marketable and more visually appealing. Is this a good thing? No, not ideally, and the best practice is to stay away from processed foods as much as possible, but this too is sometimes hard to achieve.

Comprehensive List of Food Additives to Avoid:

There are a number of definitions in the marketplace for 'Natural Food Products' and sometimes navigating the thousands of products in the grocery store aisles can be a daunting task.

Sometimes one might think that buying something that is labeled as 'Sugar-Free' or 'Fat-Free' is better for their health, when in-fact it's not. When thinking about it simply, if it comes in a packet, it's processed, and that means the food can be treated with a range of chemicals to make it look appealing and retain its shelf life. There are a few select companies that use natural ingredients like Ascorbic Acid (Vitamin C) to act as a preservative in foods, but it takes practice to find these products and typically, they are sold at health-food centered shops, rather than multinational food chains.

Essentially, limiting the consumption of processed foods is better for your health but not altogether un-avoidable. This list of additives is quite extensive, sitting at 125 of them but is another great step up from the top 12 if you want to take it even further again.

CPSIA information can be obtained
at www.ICGtesting.com
Printed in the USA
LVHW012319161220
674349LV00021B/694

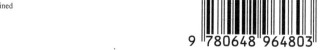